An Atlas of
DISEASES OF THE NAIL

THE ENCYCLOPEDIA OF VISUAL MEDICINE SERIES

An Atlas of
DISEASES OF THE NAIL

Phoebe Rich, MD

Oregon Health Sciences University
Portland, Oregon, USA

Richard K. Scher, MD

College of Physicians and Surgeons
Columbia University, New York, USA

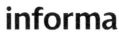

New York   London

First published in 2003 by the Parthenon Publishing Group.

This edition published in 2011 by Informa Healthcare, Telephone House, 69-77 Paul Street, London EC2A 4LQ, UK.

Simultaneously published in the USA by Informa Healthcare, 52 Vanderbilt Avenue, 7th Floor, New York, NY 10017, USA.

Informa Healthcare is a trading division of Informa UK Ltd. Registered Office: 37–41 Mortimer Street, London W1T 3JH, UK. Registered in England and Wales number 1072954.

A CIP record for this book is available from the British Library.

Library of Congress Cataloging-in-Publication Data available on application

ISBN-13: 9781850705956

Orders may be sent to: Informa Healthcare, Sheepen Place, Colchester, Essex CO3 3LP, UK
Telephone: +44 (0)20 7017 5540
Email: CSDhealthcarebooks@informa.com
Website: http://informahealthcarebooks.com/

For corporate sales please contact: CorporateBooksIHC@informa.com
For foreign rights please contact: RightsIHC@informa.com
For reprint permissions please contact: PermissionsIHC@informa.com

Contents

1

Nail anatomy and basic science

INTRODUCTION

The function of the human nail is to assist in picking up small objects, to protect the distal digit, to improve fine-touch sensation and to enhance the esthetic appearance of the hands. A complete understanding of the anatomy and physiology of the nail is essential to decipher its mysteries and its response to pathological processes.

BASIC NAIL ANATOMY AND PHYSIOLOGY

The nail is a unique structure whose component parts are collectively called the nail unit. The nail unit consists of the nail matrix, the nail bed, the hyponychium and the proximal and lateral nail folds. Anatomic structures of the nail include, from distal to proximal, the hyponychium, the onychodermal band, the nail bed, the nail plate, the lateral nail folds, the lunula, the cuticle, the nail matrix, and the proximal nail fold (Figure 1).

Nail matrix

The matrix of the nail is the germinative epithelium from which the nail plate is derived. There is controversy about whether the nail bed and nail fold contribute cells to the substance of the nail plate. Regardless of this, the matrix is responsible for the majority of the nail plate substance. The proximal portion of the matrix lies beneath the nail folds and the distal curved edge can usually be seen through the nail plate as the white lunula. The proximal matrix forms the superficial portion of the nail plate and the distal matrix makes the undersurface of the nail plate (Figure 2).

Nail bed

The nail bed dermis lies beneath the nail plate and derives its pink color from its rich vascular supply. The nail bed is sometimes called the sterile matrix and probably contributes some cells to the under-

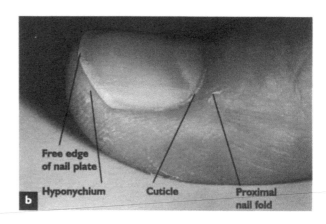

Figure 1   Anatomy of the nail. (a) Dorsal view; (b) sagittal view

surface of the nail plate, allowing the nail to grow continuously while adhering to the nail bed. Longitudinal ridges and grooves are associated with capillaries oriented in the longitudinal axis and make up the nail bed structure. This explains the orientation of splinter hemorrhages which are microhemorrhages that follow the groove in the nail bed. The nail bed extends from the nail matrix to the hyponychium. There is no subcutaneous tissue in the nail bed, so immediately beneath the nail bed lies the periostium of the distal phalanx (Figure 3).

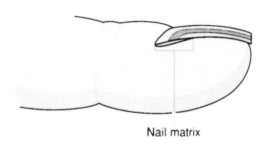

Nail matrix

Figure 2 Nail growth and production. The proximal matrix forms the superficial (dorsal) part of the nail plate. The distal nail matrix forms the ventral (underside) nail surface

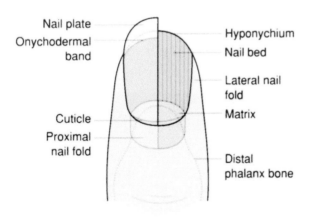

Nail plate
Onychodermal band
Cuticle
Proximal nail fold

Hyponychium
Nail bed
Lateral nail fold
Matrix
Distal phalanx bone

Figure 3 Cut-away diagram of the nail showing configuration of the nail bed and nail matrix. Note the longitudinal ridges and grooves of the nail bed. The matrix extends proximal to the proximal nail fold

Nail folds

The nail plate is surrounded by the proximal and lateral nail folds. These nail folds surround, support and protect the nail. The cuticle is the distal horny end-product of the proximal nail fold. The cuticle adheres to the nail plate and seals the nail from environmental pathogens and irritants.

Hyponychium

The hyponychium is the portion of the nail unit that is distal to the nail bed and under the free edge of the nail plate. It is contiguous with the volar skin of the digit. The hyponychium extends proximally to the distal groove and onychodermal band. The hyponychium has a granular layer unlike the matrix and nail bed, which do not.

Nail plate

The nail plate is the smooth translucent structure that is the end-product of the keratinocyte differentiation in the nail matrix. It derives its normal color appearance from the underlying structures: pink from the vascular nail bed and white from the lunula (distal part of the nail matrix) and from air under the free edge of the nail. The bulk of the nail plate comes from the nail matrix, and damage with scarring to the matrix can result in a permanent nail plate dystrophy, like a split or ridge. The surface of the nail plate is normally smooth and may develop longitudinal ridges as part of the aging process. Nail hardness is due to the disulfide bonds found in the keratin in the nail plate. The nail plate contains 0.1% calcium, although calcium contributes little to the hardness of the nail plate.

RATE OF GROWTH

Fingernails, unlike hair, grow continuously, at a rate of approximately 0.1 mm/day or 3 mm a month. Toenails grow at about one-half to one-third the rate of fingernails. A fingernail regenerates in 4–6 months, toenails in 8–12 months or more. Certain states affect the rate of nail growth; for example, nails grow faster during pregnancy and in psoriasis.

BLOOD AND NERVE SUPPLY

The nail unit has a rich blood supply. Lateral digital arteries course down the side of the digit and form arches that supply branches to the nail matrix and nail bed. During nail surgery, hemostasis can be achieved during the procedure by simply applying pressure on the sides of the digit over the digital arteries. Sensory nerves course along the sides of the digit in close association with the arteries.

FURTHER READING

Dawber RPR, de Berker DAR, Baran R. Science of the nail apparatus. In Baran R, Dawber RPR, eds. *Diseases of the Nail and Their Management*. Oxford: Blackwell Science, 1994:1–47

Fleckman P. Basic science of the nail unit. In Scher RK, Daniel CR III, eds. *Nails: Therapy, Diagnosis and Surgery*, 2nd edn. Philadelphia: WB Saunders, 1997:37–54

2

Examination of the nail and work-up of nail conditions

HISTORY

In order to accurately diagnose a nail condition, evaluation of the nail should be undertaken systematically (Table 1). A thorough history should include information about medical conditions such as anemia and endocrine disorders, dermatological history of disorders such as psoriasis, lichen planus, or alopecia areata. A history of fungal infections in other cutaneous locations, medications, occupation and hobbies may be helpful. Family history and a history of cosmetic usage should be ascertained. Was the nail condition present at birth and how has it progressed since the onset? Has it remained localized to one nail or spread to many nails? Is the problem relapsing and remitting? Is there any pain or discomfort? What treatments have been tried?

PHYSICAL EXAMINATION

Physical examination should include evaluation of all 20 nails and any concurrent skin conditions. The nails should be examined in a good light, with magnification if possible. Each component of the nail unit should be systematically evaluated, looking for changes. Are the nail beds normal? Are there changes in the hyponychium or proximal nail fold? Is there nail matrix pathology that manifests in nail plate abnormalities? The color of the nail plate and surrounding structures should be noted. If there is discoloration, is it partial or total, and what is the configuration? Is the color change due to pigment in the nail plate or in the nail bed? Are there color changes to the nail folds, capillary dilatation, erythema, melanocytic changes? Surface texture changes such as pitting, ridging, longitudinal and

Table 1 General evaluation of the patient with a nail disorder (adapted from reference 1)

History
When started, present at birth or acquired
How many nails involved (solitary nail vs multiple)
    fingernails and/or toenails
Progressive or stable
Symptomatic (painful, pruritic)
Exacerbating factors
    exposure to water, cosmetics
    trauma
What treatment has been tried

Medical history
General health, review of symptoms
Diabetes
Peripheral vascular disease, smoker, connective tissue
    disease, Raynaud's disease, arthritis

Drug history
Allergies
Anticoagulants and salicylate use

Cutaneous history
Psoriasis, lichen planus, alopecia areata, other cutaneous
    disorders with nail manifestations
Previous malignancies
Cutaneous fungal, bacterial and viral infections
Occupational history, recreation

Examination
Fingernails, toenails
Mucous membranes, hair and scalp
Pertinent cutaneous examination
Peripheral pulses in toenail disorders
Transillumination

Laboratory
X-ray imaging studies, magnetic resonance imaging
Mycology, microbiology
Histology

Photographs

horizontal grooves should be noted. Are the irregularities noted on multiple nails or a solitary nail? Do they involve the entire nail plate or are they focal? Is the perionychium intact or are there growths, irregularities, scale, color changes, vascular abnormalities, including the nail folds, hyponychium, nail bed?

LABORATORY TESTS

Appropriate laboratory tests include microscopic examination, potassium hydroxide preparation, a fungal or bacterial culture, and radiographic studies, if indicated. A potassium hydroxide preparation for the presence of fungal hyphae is quick and easy to perform and, if fungal species identification is warranted, a culture can be carried out. If fungal infection is suspected in the absence of mycologic confirmation, a nail clipping and nail bed debris or nail biopsy can be sent for histopathology and staining with PAS. These will often show the organisms. When a bacterial infection is suspected, a bacterial culture and sensitivity should be obtained so that the bacteria can be identified and appropriate antibacterial therapy can then be instituted. An X-ray and magentic resonance image of the affected digit may provide useful information in the case of a nail tumor.

NAIL BIOPSY

When history and clinical features alone do not yield a diagnosis, a biopsy of the nail should be considered. The location of the nail biopsy is dependent upon which part of the nail unit is responsible for the pathological features of the nail. When the nail plate is abnormal, the pathological process is often located in the nail matrix or is a space-occupying lesion in the nail fold. Nail bed and nail fold changes require biopsy of the appropriate area. If the clinician is not experienced or comfortable with the procedure of nail biopsy, a referral to a dermatologist should be considered (*see* Chapter 10).

FURTHER READING

Daniel CR III. An initial approach to examination of the nail. *Dermatol Clin* 1985;3:383–6

Daniel CR III. Approach to examination of the nail. In Scher RK, Daniel CR III, eds. *Nails: Therapy, Diagnosis and Surgery*. Philadelphia: WB Saunders, 1997:101–3

3

Nail signs and their definitions: non-specific nail dystrophies

The nail is limited in its response to pathological processes. An understanding of these non-specific nail findings helps with the diagnosis and differential diagnosis of nail conditions. When the abnormal features are identified correctly, a differential diagnosis can be generated. Most of the common nail findings will be illustrated with clues to the proper diagnosis. The location of the pathological process in the nail unit is not always the site of the morphological nail finding. It is important to consider the origin of the finding so that therapy is directed to the correct site. For example, pitting must be treated at the level of the nail matrix. It is useless to treat the nail plate for pitting because the pathology that causes pitting is in the matrix.

The nail plate is the end-product of the nail matrix and, in its normal state, is a smooth translucent hard structure that is tightly adherent to the nail bed. Nail plate abnormalities can be traced to the nail matrix, as in pitting, or to the nail bed or nail fold, as in a space-occupying lesion.

ANONYCHIA

Anonychia is the absence of nail. It can occur as the end result of scarring (onychatrophy) (Figure 4) and in congenital disorders, often when there is malformation of the corresponding digit (Figure 5).

BEAU'S LINES

Beau's lines are horizontal grooves in the nail plate that represent an arrest or slow-down in the growth of the nail matrix. A severe medical event such as surgery, allergic reaction to medication or serious trauma to the system can trigger Beau's lines. The depth and width of the line speak to the abruptness

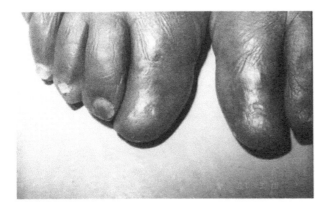

Figure 4   Anonychia or absence of the nail as a result of lichen planus

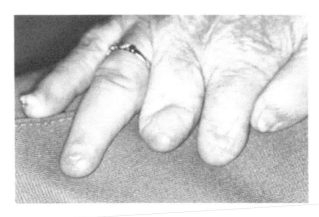

Figure 5   Congenital anonychia

and duration of the event. Beau's lines move distally as the nail grows over time (Figure 6).

BRACHYONYCHIA

In brachyonychia, or short nails, the longitudinal dimension of the nail is shorter than normal, giving the fingernail an unusually broad appearance. This can occur as an isolated finding and there may be shortening of the terminal phalanx. The thumbs are commonly affected (racket nails) and this may be familial (Figures 7 and 8).

CHROMONYCHIA

Chromonychia is the presence of abnormal nail color. The natural nail plate is translucent and derives its apparent color from the underlying structures. Certain internal diseases and medications can cause color abnormalities in the nail plate. External factors can stain and discolor the nail plate. When the pigmentation is caused by external factors, the change in pigmentation parallels the contour of the proximal nail fold and, when caused by internal factors, the change usually follows the lunula contour.

CLUBBING

Clubbing is present when there are both increased curvature of the nail in the horizontal axis and a bulbous overgrowth of the tip of the digit. The most common cause of acquired clubbing is pulmonary disorders (Figure 9) (*see* Chapter 7 for more information on clubbing).

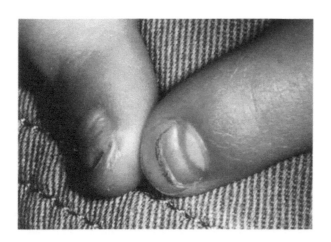

Figure 6   Beau's lines resulting from growth arrest of the nail matrix

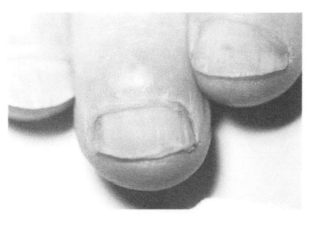

Figure 7   Shortened nails/brachyonychia

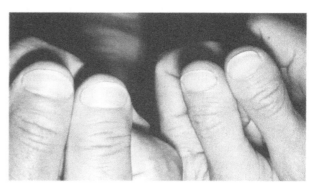

Figure 8   Familial racket nail of the thumb in father and daughter

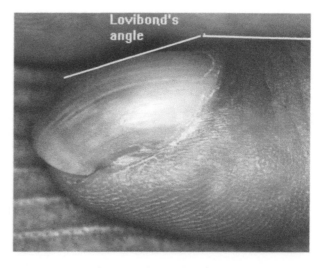

Figure 9   Clubbing, with Lovibond's angle greater than 180°

HABIT TIC DEFORMITY

Habit tic deformity has the appearance of parallel horizontal grooves in the nail plate, as the result of repetitive minor trauma to the proximal nail plate and lunula. The defect formed by the chronic picking and rubbing and the grooved appearance of the nail have been described as resembling a washboard. Thumbs are most commonly involved and the lunula is usually enlarged. The nail often grows in normally when the chronic picking ceases (Figures 10 and 11).

KOILONYCHIA

Koilonychia occurs when the free edge of the nail is everted, resulting in a concave 'spoon nail'. There are many causes of koilonychia ranging from anemia and thyroid abnormalities to a normal finding in some children (Figure 12) (*see* Chapter 7).

LEUKONYCHIA

Leukonychia is the name given to white nails. The condition can be congenital or acquired, complete or

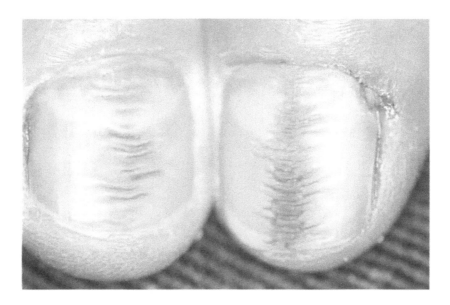

Figure 10   Habit tic deformity

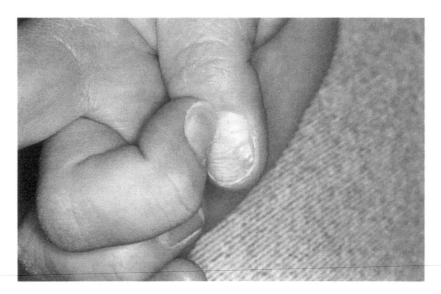

Figure 11   Habit tic deformity

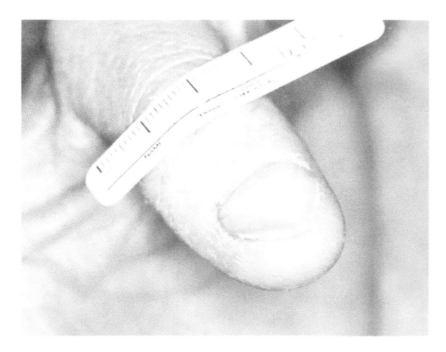

Figure 12   Koilonychia

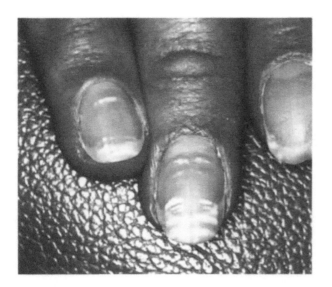

Figure 13   Punctate and transverse leukonychia

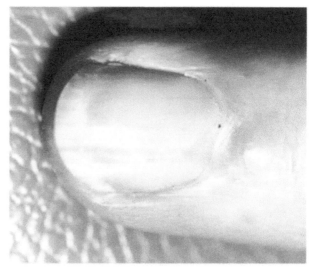

Figure 14   Myxoid cyst in proximal nail fold causing a nail plate deformity

partial, and true or apparent (*see* Chapter 4 for more thorough discussion of leukonychia). Punctate and striate leukonychia (Figure 13) is a common partial leukonychia. It is due to microtrauma of the matrix near the proximal nail fold that causes parakeratotic cells to form in the nail plate. These white spots grow out with the nail.

LONGITUDINAL GROOVES

Longitudinal depressions can occur in the nail as a result of a space-occupying lesion in the nail fold overlying the nail matrix. The mass presses on the matrix and nascent nail resulting in a depressed deformity. Lesions such as myxoid cyst (Figure 14) and fibroma (Figure 15) can cause the groove. When the mass is removed, the nail usually grows in normally (*see* myxoid cyst).

and Maffuci's syndrome. It may also be seen in tumors of the distal phalanx such as osteochondroma.

MACRONYCHIA

Macronychia is the name for large nails. These can occur in patients with congenital abnormalities like macrodactyly as in Proteus syndrome (Figure 16)

MEDIAN NAIL DYSTROPHY

Median nail dystrophy (of Heller)[1] is an unusual condition of unknown etiology that causes a linear deformity and split in the mid-line of the nail,

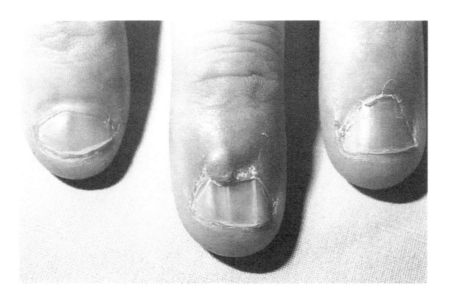

Figure 15   Fibroma causing nail plate grooves

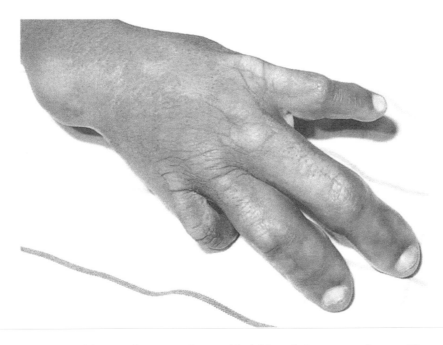

Figure 16   Macronychia in an 8-year-old child with Proteus syndrome. The nails of the affected digit are significantly larger than those of the unaffected hand

usually of the thumb. It can resemble an inverse chevron or fir-tree pattern (Figure 17). The defect is usually self-healing, but may be recurrent.

MELANONYCHIA STRIATA

Melanonychia striata, also called longitudinal melanonychia, is characterized by longitudinal,

pigmented bands of the nails. There are many benign causes of melanonychia including nevi, lentigines, drugs and trauma, but the most important differential diagnosis is malignant melanoma of the nail (Figures 18 and 19) (*see* Chapters 4 and 9).

MICRONYCHIA

Micronychia means small nails. It is usually due to a congenital defect (Figure 20). Congenital onychodystrophy of the index finger (COIF syndrome) is a rare syndrome of unknown prevalence in which there is dystrophy of the index fingernail and often the underlying bone[2,3].

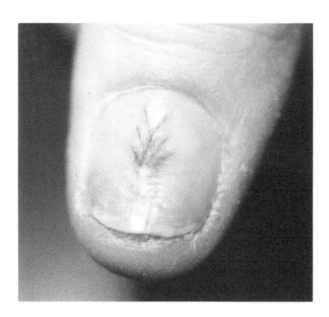

Figure 17　Median nail dystrophy

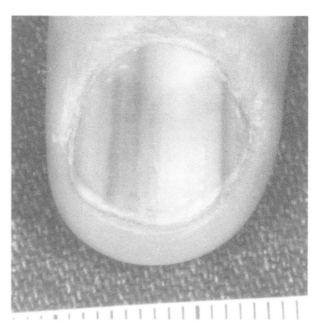

Figure 19　Melanoma *in situ*

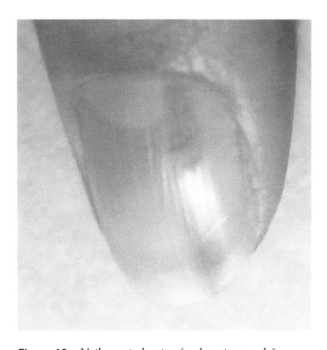

Figure 18　Nail matrix lentigo (melanotic macule)

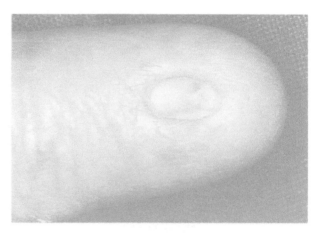

Figure 20　Small nail in idiopathic micronychia

ONYCHATROPHY

Onychatrophy is atrophic loss of the nails, often following a scarring process that irreversibly scars the nail matrix to prevent growth of the nail plate. Onychotillomania is the compulsive picking of the nail and can result in onychatrophy in severe cases (Figure 21).

ONYCHOGRYPHOSIS

Onychogryphosis occurs when the nail plate becomes hyperkeratotic and grossly thickened. The nail may curve as it thickens. It is due to hypertrophy of the nail plate and can appear as a ram's horn dystrophy. It occurs most commonly in the toe nails of elderly people with biomechanical problems or the inability to groom the nails properly or with poorly fitting footwear (Figure 22). The thickened nails may become painful. It can be associated with psoriasis, impaired peripheral circulation and neglect. Less commonly, onychogryphosis involves the finernails (Figure 23).

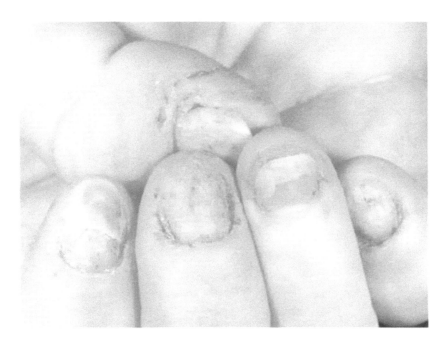

Figure 21 Onychotillomania and onychatrophy due to chronic picking and tearing of the nails

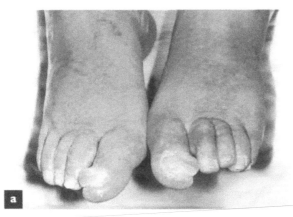
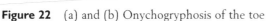
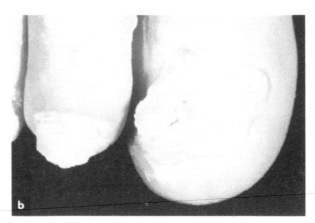

Figure 22 (a) and (b) Onychogryphosis of the toe

ONYCHOMADESIS

Onychomadesis is shedding of the nails. This process begins in the proximal area, usually related to a systemic insult that causes a growth arrest. The nail is shed and is usually replaced by a normal nail, although there can be permanent loss if there is severe scarring in the nail matix. Medications such as chemotherapy agents for cancer[4], viral infections, pemphigus vulgaris and casting for fracture have been associated with onychomadesis (Figure 24) (for more information, *see* Chapter 8).

ONYCHORRHEXIS

Onychorrhexis is defined as longitudinal ridging of the nail plate and can be seen in several nail conditions such as lichen planus (Figure 25), Darier's disease, and circulatory disorders (Figure 26). Longitudinal ridges can be seen as a normal phenomenon in nails of the elderly (Figure 27). Often, there are small chips at the free edge in the troughs between the ridges, where the nail is fragile.

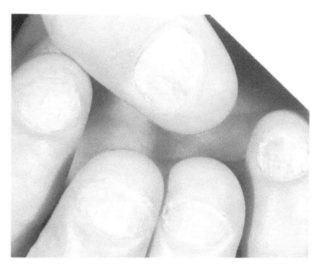

Figure 25   Onychorrhexis due to lichen planus

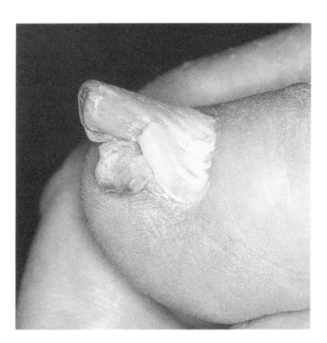

Figure 23   Onychogryphosis of the finger

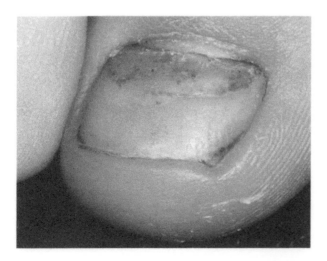

Figure 24   Onychomadesis in a child due to medications

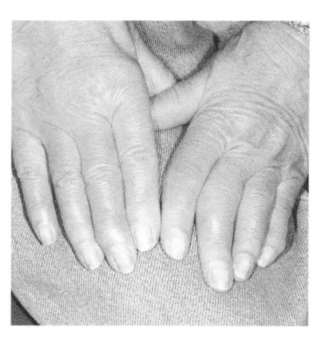

Figure 26   Onychorrhexis in Raynaud's disease

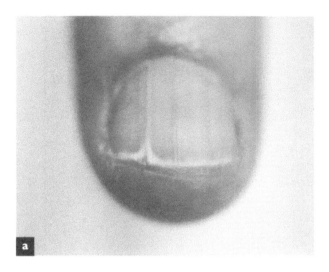

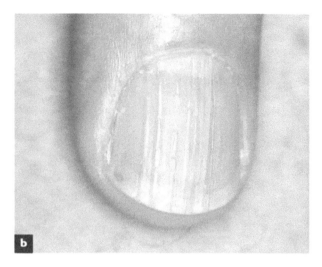

Figure 27 (a) and (b) Onychorrhexis: longitudinal ridges and splits in aging nails

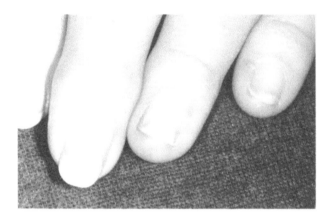

Figure 28 Onycholysis is separation of the nail plate from the nail bed and occurs in many settings including psoriasis

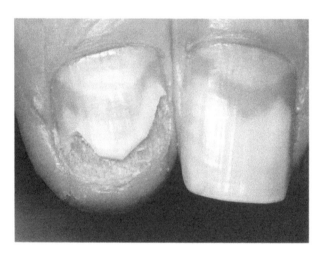

Figure 29 Onycholysis, with separation of the nail plate from the nail bed. Affected areas appear white because there is air beneath the nail plate

ONYCHOLYSIS

Onycholysis is defined as the separation of the nail plate from the underlying nail bed[5]. It occurs when the distal attachment of the nail plate to the nail bed is disrupted by trauma, water, or nail bed disease (Figure 28). Onycholysis begins distally with a disruption of the distal attachment of the nail plate to the nail bed. The onycholytic portion of the nail appears white because there is air beneath the nail plate (Figure 29). Onycholysis is associated with psoriasis (Figure 30), onychomycosis, yellow nail syndrome, contact dermatitis, medications and endocrine disorders, as well as many environmental causes.

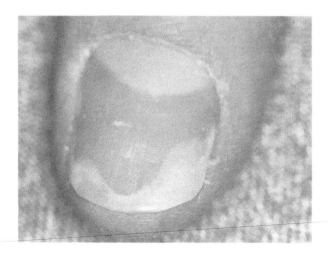

Figure 30 Onycholysis in psoriasis

Onycholysis can be drug-induced, as in photo-onycholysis (Figure 31) attributed to doxycycline, and it can be self-induced (Figure 32). Once the separation of the nail plate from the nail bed occurs, the space created beneath the loosened nail plate can become secondarily infected by microorganisms, particularly *Candida albicans* and *Pseudomonas* (Figure 33). These infections often perpetuate the onycholysis. Protecting the affected nail from water exposure and trauma will often allow the nail bed to heal. If *Candida* is present, appropriate antifungal medications should be employed. Occasionally, a staphylococcal infection occurs under the onycholytic nail, at which time the drainage should be cultured and antibiotics given (Figure 34). Neglected subungual bacterial infection can result in osteomyelitis (Figure 35).

If chronic unexplained onycholysis is present, the possibility of subungual squamous cell carcinoma should be considered and a biopsy performed (Figure 36).

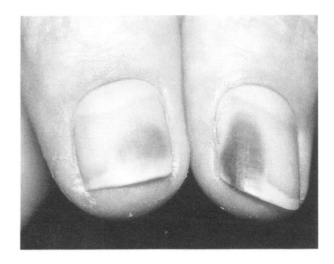

Figure 33 Secondary infection by *Pseudomonas* in onycholysis

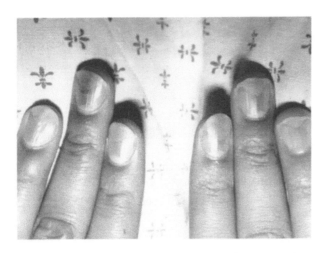

Figure 31 Photo-onycholysis in drug-induced onycholysis

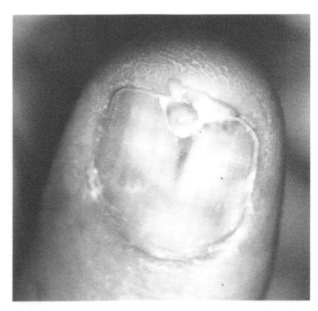

Figure 34 *Staphylococcal* infection under the onycholytic nail

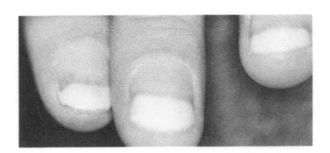

Figure 32 Self-induced onycholysis

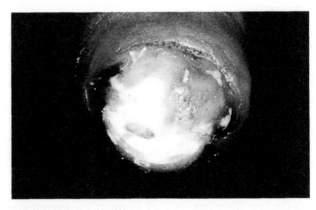

Figure 35 Osteomyelitis

ONYCHOSCHIZIA

Onychoschizia is characterized by distal peeling and lamellar separation of the layers of the nail plate at the free edge. This makes the nail fragile and subject to chipping and fractures. Under experimental conditions, 21 days of alternate wetting and dehydration caused onychoschizia. Irritants, detergents and excessive water exposure exacerbate this condition, while moisturizing may provide some relief.

The B vitamin, Biotin 2500 μg daily, has been shown to be helpful with brittle nails and onychoschizia (Figures 37 and 38).

PACHYONYCHIA

Pachyonychia is defined as thick nails as in the autosomal dominant condition of pachyonychia congenita (Figure 39) (*see* Chapter 8).

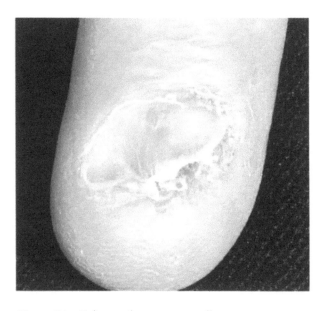

Figure 36 Subungual squamous cell carcinoma *in situ* associated with onycholysis. Part of the onycholytic nail has been cut away

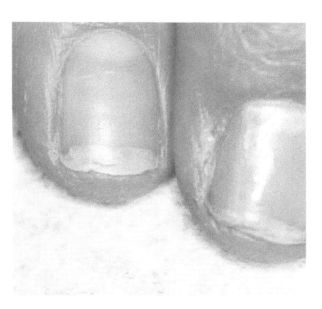

Figure 38 Onychoschizia, with distal peeling, layering and splitting of the nail plate

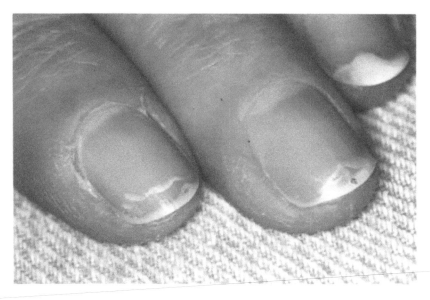

Figure 37 Onychoschizia

PARONYCHIA

The perionychium consists of the proximal and lateral nail folds[8] (Figure 40). Paronychia is inflammation and/or infection of these folds. It can be acute bacterial paronychia (Figure 41) or a chronic paronychia (Figure 42) that is primarily irritant or allergic but may be secondarily infected with *Candida*[9].

Acute paronychia

Acute paronychia is usually due to *Staphylococcus* and presents with a painful, red, warm nail fold. There may be pus present (Figure 43), which should be cultured so that appropriate antibiotics can be administered. The inciting event in acute paronychia is injury to, or disruption of, the cuticle and nail folds (Figure 44) which opens a portal for infection. Ingrown toenails can precipitate an acute paronychia,

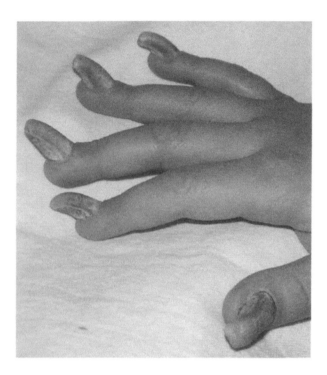

Figure 39   Pachyonychia congenita

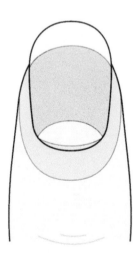

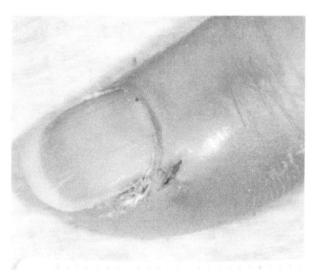

Figure 41   Acute paronychia is usually due to *Staphylococcal* bacteria

Figure 40   The perionychium consists of the proximal and lateral nail folds. In the diagram, the shaded area indicates the perionychium

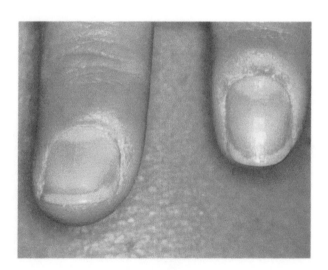

Figure 42   Chronic paronychia

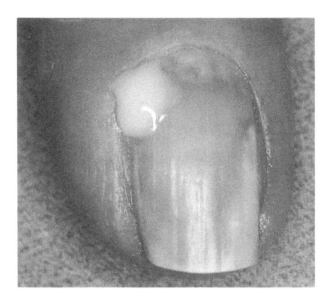

Figure 43 Acute paronychia with pus present in the infected nail fold

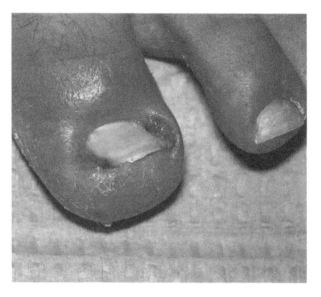

Figure 44 Ingrown toenail causing acute paronychia caused by *Staphylococcal* infection. Granulation tissue and pyogenic granuloma are present

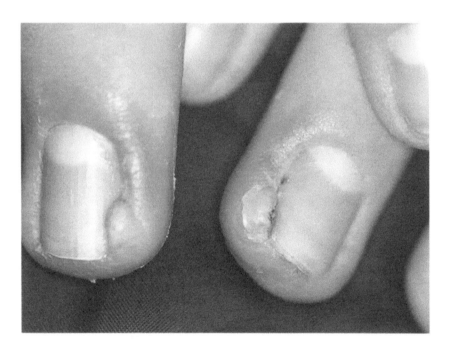

Figure 45 Paronychia associated with oral retinoid therapy

and paronychia is sometimes associated with oral retinoid therapy (Figure 45).

Chronic paronychia

Chronic paronychia usually starts from trauma or irritant reaction from exposure to environmental irritants or foods. Housewives, cooks, waitresses and other people with wet work jobs are at risk for chronic paronychia (Figure 46). With the cuticle gone, the potential space under the nail fold is open to contamination with ubiquitous yeasts and bacteria. The nail fold becomes swollen and inflamed (Figure 47). As the chronic paronychia progresses, the nail plate develops horizontal ridges and grooves (Figure 48). The treatment includes removal of the

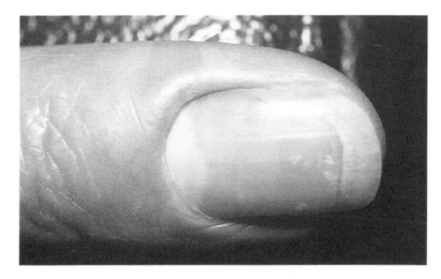

Figure 46   Chronic paronychia from contact irritants

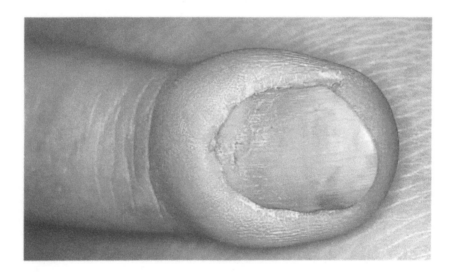

Figure 47   Inflamed nail fold in chronic paronychia

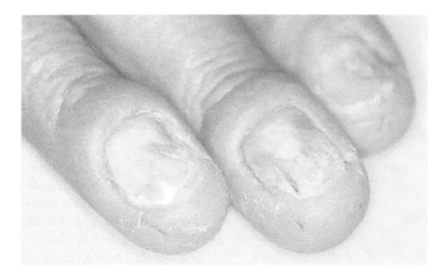

Figure 48   Chronic paronychia resulting in nail plate changes

environmental factors and allergens that triggered the problem and treatment of yeast and bacteria, when present. Once the cuticle and nail fold heal themselves, the nail plate will regain its smooth surface. In some cases, topical and intralesional corticosteroids are helpful[10].

PINCER NAIL

Pincer nail describes an exaggerated transverse over-curvature of the nail plate along the longitudinal axis (Figures 49 and 50). Pincer nails are usually acquired during advancing age but occasionally are congenital. There is often enlargement of the underlying bony phalanx. Sometimes, the nail curves into the nail fold and nail bed, causing pain and infection. Avulsion of the nail plate does not correct the underlying problem because the underlying bone and nail bed are misshapen, so the nail will grow back as bad or worse than before the surgery[11]. The best approach is to remove the lateral portion of the nail matrix surgically or with chemical destruction with phenol (*see* Chapter 10).

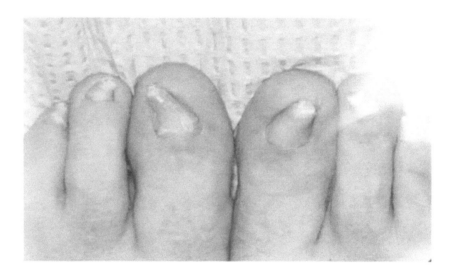

Figure 49   Pincer nail

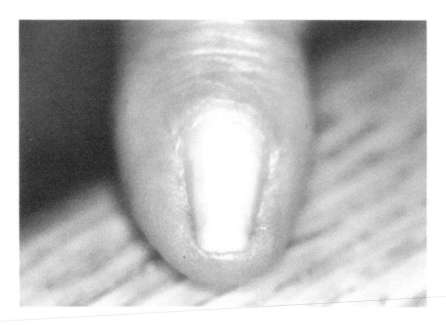

Figure 50   Pincer nail

PITTING

Nail pits are small, round depressions on the surface of the nail plate. They are usually due to disease in the proximal matrix or, sometimes, the proximal nail fold. Nail pitting can be seen in psoriasis, alopecia areata, and eczema. Random pits in the nail can be seen as an isolated idiopathic finding. Pitting in psoriatic nails occurs when small foci of psoriatic hyperkeratosis indent the nascent nail and then fall away after the area grows past the proximal nail fold.

The configuration of nail pitting depends on the area of the matrix involved, and the duration of the pathological process in the nail matrix. The longitudinal dimension of the pits is determined by the length of time that the psoriasis is active in that portion of the nail matrix (Figure 51).

The arrangement of the depressions in the surface of the nail can be in regular or in haphazard arrays. Pitting seen in psoriasis and alopecia areata, presumably due to the extent and location of the disease in the nail matrix, can be confluent or, more commonly, is scattered, although in alopecia areata a linear arrangement often occurs (Figure 52). When the pitting is uniformly distributed, giving the entire nail plate a roughened appearance, it is called trachyonychia (*see* section on trachyonychia). Pitting is sometimes seen in severe eczema that affects the proximal nail folds. The changes can be intermittent, giving the appearance of parallel horizontal depressions corresponding to the waxing and waning course of eczema. Treatment of pitting due to any of the dermatological disorders must be directed to the matrix of the nail. Topical corticosteroids under occlusion and intralesional triamcinolone acetonide 2–3 mg/ml into the proximal nail fold are the most effective treatment for nail pitting.

PTERYGIUM

Dorsal pterygium is a scarring process where there is thinning and atrophy of the nail plate, with eventual growth of the proximal nail fold onto the nail bed (Figure 53). The scarring can involve the matrix and result in total permanent scarring of the nail. It is seen in advanced lichen planus, peripheral vascular disease, and injury of the nail. Ventral pterygium occurs when the distal nail bed and hyponychium attach to the under surface of the nail plate.

Ventral or inverse pterygium occurs when the hyponychium tissue grows and attaches to the

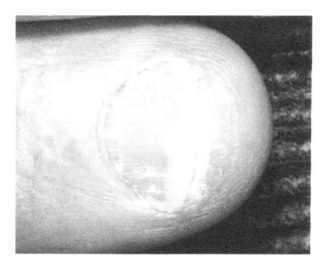

Figure 51   Pitting in psoriasis

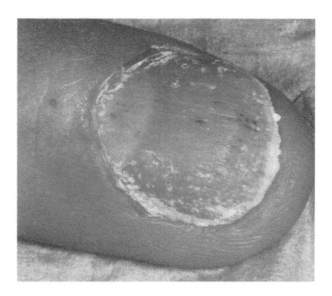

Figure 52   Pitting is characteristic of nail matrix psoriasis. Note also the splinter hemorrhages, which are due to nail bed psoriasis

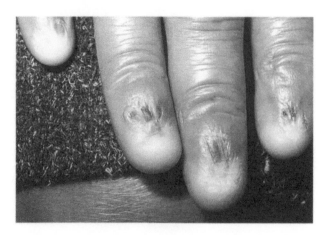

Figure 53   Dorsal pterygium

ventral surface of the nail plate. Ventral pterygium can be seen in people with connective tissue disorders such as scleroderma (Figure 54) and systemic lupus erythematosus. Ventral pterygium can be familial or idiopathic. There may be nail fold capillary prominence associated with ventral pterygium in patients with connective tissue disease.

SPLINTER HEMORRHAGES

Splinter hemorrhages appear as thin, longitudinal, red–brown lines that resemble splinters under the nail plate. The configuration of splinter hemorrhages is due to the longitudinal grooves of the nail bed collecting microscopic hemorrhages. Most splinter hemorrhages are located in the distal third of the nail. The most common cause of splinter hemorrhages is trauma. Psoriasis and other medical and vascular events have been associated with the appearance of splinter hemorrhages in the nail[12] (Figure 55).

SUBUNGUAL HEMORRHAGE

When an injury to the nail occurs, a hemorrhage often forms under the nail plate (Figure 56). This

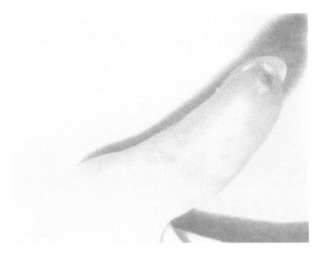

Figure 54 Inverse pterygium in a patient with scleroderma (systemic sclerosis)

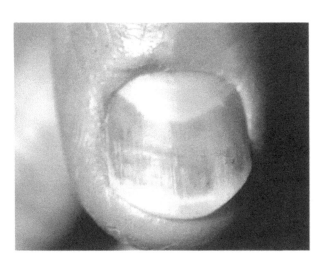

Figure 55 Splinter hemorrhage in psoriasis

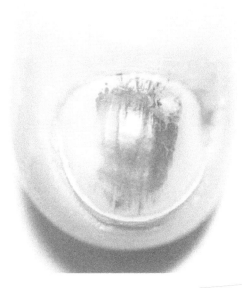

Figure 56 Subungual hemorrhage due to intralesional cortisone injections for psoriasis

blue/black lesion usually grows out with the nail. The important issue with subungual hemorrhage is that it needs to be distinguished from subungual melanocytic lesions, especially melanoma. Any persistent hemorrhage needs to be biopsied in order to be certain that the pigment is due to blood. Often, the nail plate overlying the hemorrhage is not attached and can be clipped away (Figure 57).

TRACHYONYCHIA

Trachyonychia is the term for an irregular surface of the nail plate that is composed of small irregular pitting and gives the nail a roughened, lusterless surface (Figure 58). Trachyonychia has been termed 20-nail dystrophy of childhood[13,14]. This term is a slight misnomer because the condition occurs in

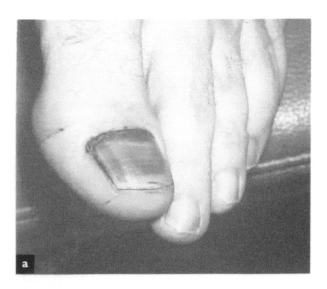
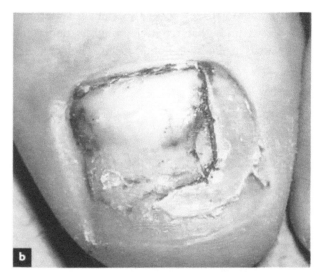

Figure 57 (a) and (b) Nail hemorrhage with cutting of nail plate

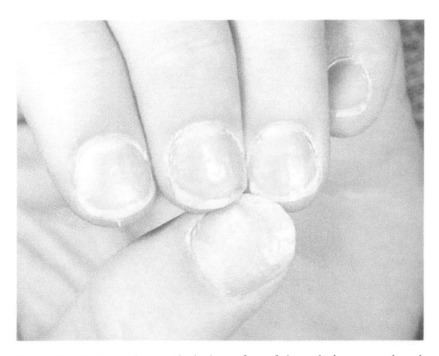

Figure 58 Trachyonychia in which the surface of the nail plate is rough and appears dull and lusterless

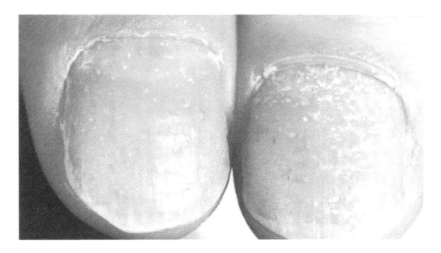

Figure 59 Trachyonychia in alopecia areata

adults as well as children, and one to 20 nails may be affected. In children, trachyonychia sometimes resolves spontaneously. Trachyonychia is associated with alopecia areata (Figure 59), psoriasis, lichen planus, chronic eczema and ichthyosis vulgaris, as well as other conditions.

REFERENCES

1. Rehtijarva K. Dystrophica mediana canaliformis (Heller). *Acta Dermatol Venerol* 1971;51:315

2. Miura T, Nakamura R. Congenital onychodysplasia of the index fingers. *J Hand Surg [Am]* 1990;15:793–7

3. Prais D, Merlob P, Horey G. COIF syndrome: the diversity of clinical and radiological findings. *Am J Med Genet* 2002;107:179–80

4. Cetin M, Utas S, Unal, A, Altimbas M. Shedding of the nails due to chemotherapy (onychomadesis). *J Eur Acad Dermatol Venereol* 1998;11:193–4

5. Daniel CR III. Onycholysis: an overview. *Semin Dermatol* 1991;10:34–40

6. Wallace MS, Bowen WR, Guinn JD. Pathogenesis of onychoschizia (lamellar dystrophy). *J Am Acad Dermatol* 1991;24:44–8

7. Colombo VE, Gerber F, Bronhofer M, Floersheim GL. Treatment of brittle fingernails and onychoschizia with biotin: scanning electron microscopy. *J Am Acad Dermatol* 1990;23:1127–32

8. Zook EG. Understanding the perionychium. *J Hand Ther* 2000;13:269–75

9. Daniel CR, Gupta AK, Daniel MP, Sullivan S. Candida infection of the nail: role of Candida as a primary or secondary pathogen. *Int J Dermatol* 1998;37:904–7

10. Tosti A, Piraccini BM, Ghetti E, Colomubo MD. Topical steroids versus systemic antifungals in the treatment of chronic paronychia: An open, randomized double-blind and double dummy study. *J Am Acad Dermatol* 2002;47:73–6

11. Baran R, Haneke E, Richert B. Pincer nails: definition and surgical treatment. *Dermatol Surg* 2001;27:261–6

12. Mujicc F, Lloyd M, Caudrado MJ, Khamashta MA, Hughes, GR. Prevalence and clinical significance of subungual splinter haemorrhages in patients with the antiphospholipid syndrome. *Clin Exp Rheumatol* 1995;13:327–31

13. Taniguchi S, Kutsuna H, Tani Y, Kawahiraa K, Hamada T. Twenty-nail dystrophy (trachyonychia) caused by lichen planus in a patient with alopecia universalis and ichthyosis vulgaris. *J Am Acad Dermatol* 1995;33:903–5

14. Tosti A, Bardazzi F, Piraccini BM, Fanti, PA. Idiopathic trachyonychia (twenty-nail dystrophy): a pathological study of 23 patients. *Br J Dermatol* 1994;131:866–72

4

Chromonychias

Chromonychia or changes in nail color can be due to exogenous causes, infectious agents, internal disorders and abnormalities of nail melanocyte proliferation or melanin production. It is helpful to consider nail dyschromia according to color.

LEUKONYCHIA (WHITE NAILS)

The term leukonychia is used to describe nails that appear white. It can be divided into several categories: partial versus complete, true versus apparent, and congenital versus acquired.

True leukonychia occurs when the actual nail plate is white due to alterations of the nail plate keratinocytes. Apparent leukonychia is due to alterations in the nail bed, matrix or hyponychium that give the nail the white appearance.

Punctate leukonychia is common and results from minor nail trauma to the nail in the vicinity of the nail matrix, resulting in nucleated keratinocytes in the nail, which appear as small white areas (Figure 60). An extension of punctate leukonychia is transverse leukonychia, also due to trauma to the matrix, often during manicuring. These narrow white lines

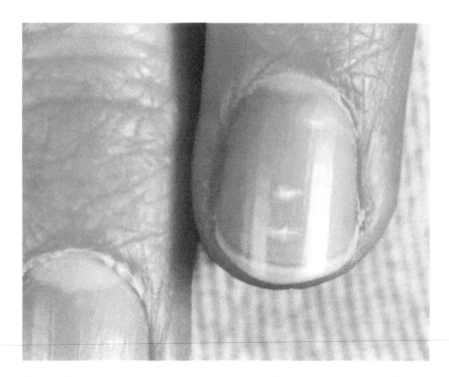

Figure 60   Punctate leukonychia with nucleated keratinocytes in the nail plate

are often parallel with the proximal nail fold and grow out with the nail. True leukonychia can be seen in some types of onychomycosis and psoriasis.

Apparent leukonychia describes a nail that looks white but is, in fact, normal in color. Onycholysis is an example of apparent leukonychia because the white appearance is due to air beneath the nail. When the nail is removed in apparent leukonychia, the nail plate is of normal color (Figure 61). Three examples of pseudoleukonychia are Terry's nail, Muehrche's lines, and half-and-half nails. These conditions are due to nail bed whitening.

Terry's nails (Figure 62) appear milky white and opaque from the lunula to the onychodermal band. Terry's nails are seen in patients with hepatic dysfunction and cirrhosis. There have been reports of Terry's nails in patients with chronic congestive heart disease, type 2 diabetes mellitus, and aging. The Terry's nails of congestive heart failure may also be pink, a different presentation from the white nails of liver disease.

Muehrche's lines (Figure 63) are white horizontal bands that are parallel to the lunula and separated by pink bands. This condition occurs when the serum

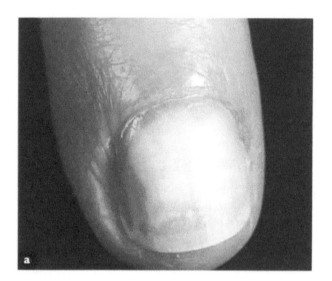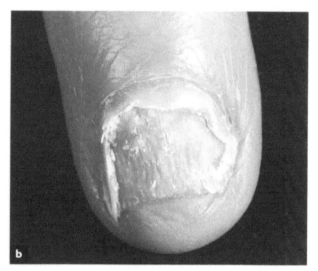

Figure 61 Apparent leukonychia caused by onycholysis. (a) White appearance of nail due to air beneath the nail plate; (b) the nail plate is of normal color when the nail is removed

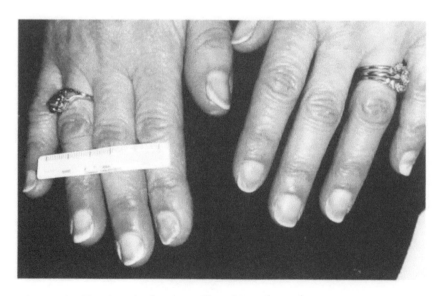

Figure 62 Terry's nails, showing milky white color and opaqueness

albumin is low, and disappears when the albumin levels return to normal. Muehrche's lines occur in patients with renal failure and/or hemodialysis.

The half-and-half nail has a proximal, opaque, white portion that obscures the lunula and a distal red/brown color (Figure 64). It also occurs in patients in renal failure and on hemodialysis.

Other causes of true leukonychia are onychomycosis and psoriasis.

YELLOW NAILS

In the yellow nail syndrome, the nail changes are characterized by yellow, slow-growing nails with absent lunula and cuticle (Figure 65). Yellow nail syndrome is usually associated with a pulmonary problem such as pleural effusion, bronchiectasis or chronic sinus infection. The underlying pathological process is thought to be related to impaired lymphatic drainage.

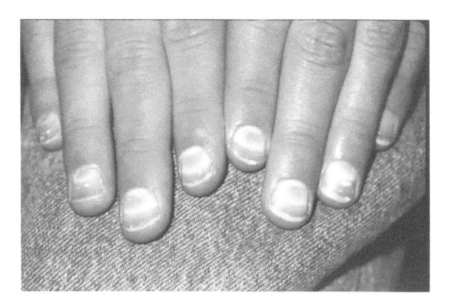

Figure 63 Muehrche's nails in a patient with low serum albumin

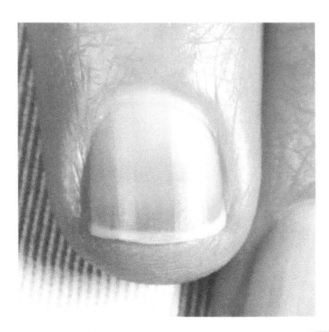

Figure 64 Half-and-half nails in patient with renal failure

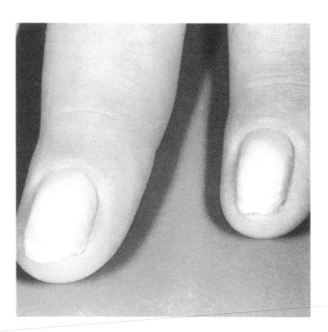

Figure 65 Yellow nail syndrome, with opaque yellow nails, absent lunula and cuticle

Yellow nails can be caused by staining of the nail plate by prolonged usage of nail enamel. The nail plate is stained by the dye in nail polish (Figure 66). Some medications, including tetracycline, can cause a yellow discoloration of the nail.

BLUE NAILS

Blue nails can result from medications such as minocycline (Figure 67), antimalarials, phenothalein,

bleomycin, and phenothiazines. Wilson's disease and argyria (Figure 68) can be associated with blue nails.

RED NAILS

The normal color of the nail bed is light red or pink. There are some pathologic processes where a portion of the nail unit is red. Red spots in the lunula (Figures 69 and 70) are seen in several disorders including psoriasis, lichen planus, alopecia areata. Diffuse reddish lunula are seen with systemic lupus, rheumatoid arthritis, cardiac disease and others.

Glomus tumor (see Figure 173) is seen as a red macule beneath the nail. Carbon monoxide poisoning, systemic lupus erythematosus and polycythemia cause red changes in the nail unit.

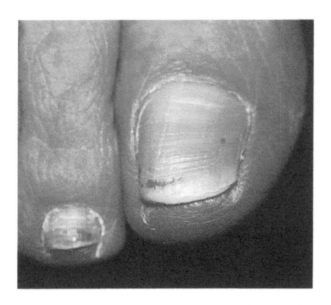

Figure 66   Yellow staining of the nail plate from the dye in nail enamel

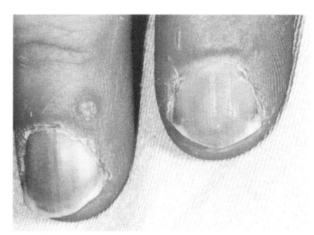

Figure 68   Blue band in the nail caused by argyria

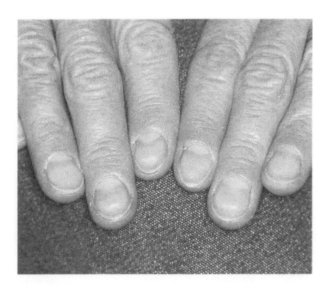

Figure 67   Blue discoloration of the nail from minocycline

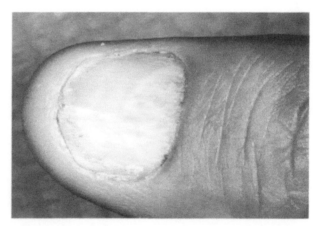

Figure 69   Red spots in the lunula

BROWN–BLACK PIGMENTATION OF THE NAIL

Brown–black pigmentation of the nail is termed melanonychia. Melanonychia can be diffuse or partial, taking the form of longitudinal brown bands in the nail plate. The most important cause of longitudinal pigmentation of the nail is subungual melanoma, although there are many benign causes of longitudinal melanonychia. Melanonychia is due to melanin, as in nevi (Figure 71), lentigos and melanoma. Melanoma can begin as a longitudinal pigmented band in the nail plate or, less frequently, in the nail bed. There may be the Hutchinson's sign where there is spread of pigment onto the nail folds. Benign melanonychia can be caused by drugs (Figure 72), vitamin B12 deficiencies (Figure 73), and Laugier–Huntziger syndrome in which there are pigmented bands in the nails and pigmented macules on the lips and mucosa (Figures 74 and 75). Melanonychia striata can be seen as a normal finding

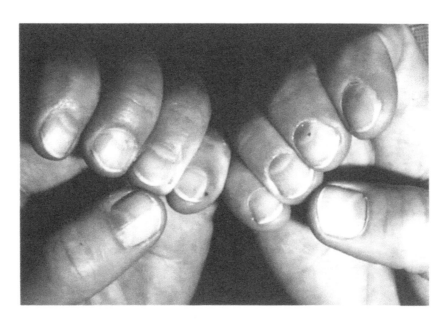

Figure 70   Red lunula

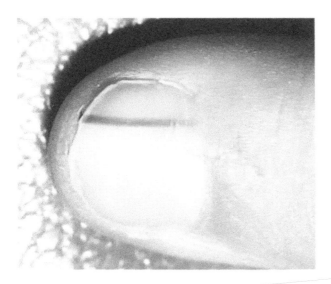

Figure 71   Melanonychia due to a nail matrix nevus

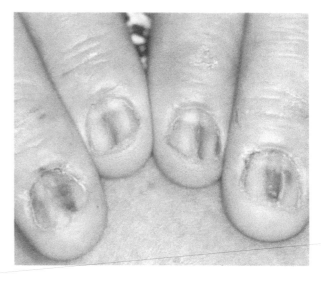

Figure 72   Benign melanonychia caused by zidovudine

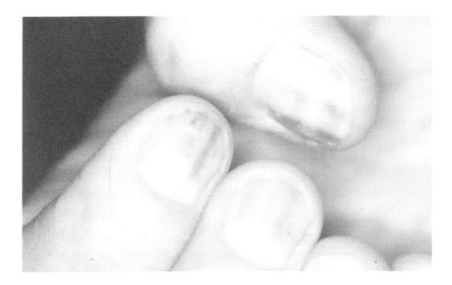

Figure 73 Melanonychia caused by vitamin B12 deficiency

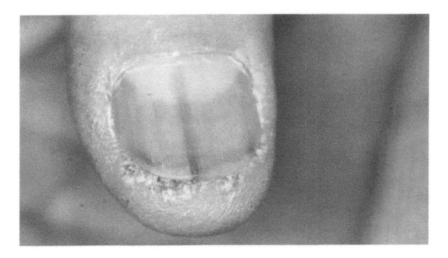

Figure 74 Laugier–Huntziger syndrome with longitudinal melanonychia and mucosal melanotic macules

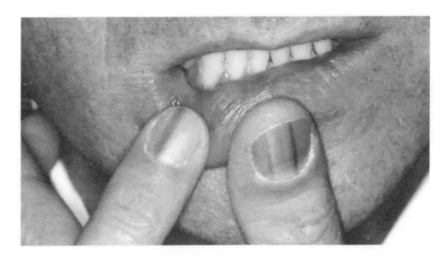

Figure 75 Laugier–Huntziger syndrome

in darkly pigmented individuals. If the diagnosis is in question, a biopsy of the nail is mandatory (Figure 76). Table 2 lists the causes of melanonychia.

EXOGENOUS NAIL DYSCHROMIA

Nail dyschromia can be the result of exogenous pigment in the nail. Pigments and stains in the workplace and home can be deposited on the surface of the nail. Exogenous dyschromia is easily recognized because the proximal border of the discoloration is parallel to the proximal nail fold. The proximal margin of internally caused dyschromia is usually parallel to the lunula (Figures 77 and 78).

ERYTHRONYCHIA

Longitudinal erythronychia, a clinical entity well known for many years among dermatologists with an interest in nail disorders, was recently described by Baran and Perrin (Figure 79). In their series of 16 cases, they found that 14 were onychopapillomas, but two turned out on biopsy to be Bowen's disease. Therefore, the latter condition should at least be considered in the differential diagnosis. The clinical features include an erythematous band of the nail bed which was sometimes associated with splinter hemorrhages and distal subungual hyperkeratosis.

Table 2 Causes of pigmentation in the nail. Reproduced with permission from Lawry M, Rich P. *Current Problems in Dermatology* 1999;11:161–208

Melanin and melanin complexes
Normal variant for skin phototype IV, V and VI**
Hypermelanosis of the matrix epithelium (melanotic macule equivalent)
Lentigenous melanocytic hyperplasia*
Junctional nevus*
Compound nevus*
Malignant melanoma*
Bowen's disease, squamous cell carcinoma, basal cell carcinoma*
Laugier–Huntziger syndrome/Peutz–Jegher syndrome**
Addison's disease, Cushing's syndrome**
Post-inflammatory hyperpigmentation (i.e. lichen planus, trauma)†
Drugs (AZT, antimetabolites, antimalarials, minocycline)**
Heavy metal exposure**

Non-melanin pigmentation
Demateacious fungi†
Bacteria (pseudomonas)†
Hematoma (hemoglobin/hemosiderin)*

*Most commonly seen in one digit; **most commonly seen in multiple digits; †can be seen in single or multiple digits

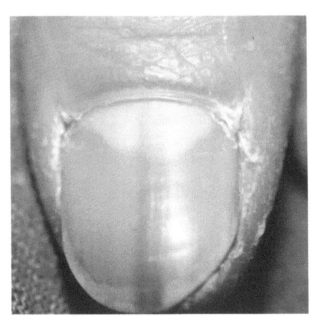

Figure 76 Nail matrix lentigo (melanotic macule)

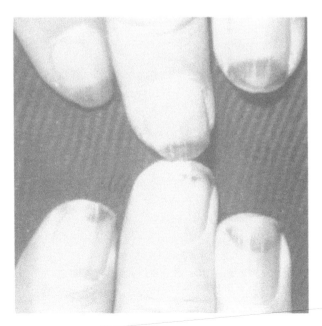

Figure 77 Exogenous pigment in nail plate from shelling walnuts

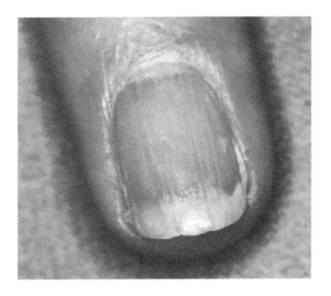

Figure 78   Yellow staining of nail plate from nail polish

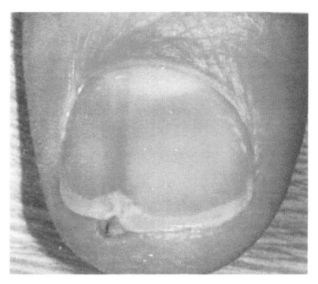

Figure 79   Erythronychia

FURTHER READING

Grossman M, Scher RK. Leukonychia: review and classification. *Int J Dermatol* 1990;29:535–41

Baran R, Perrin C. Longitudinal erythronychia with distal subungual keratosis: onychopapilloma of the nail bed and Bowen's disease. *Br J Dermatol* 2000;143:132–5

Daniel CR III. Nail pigment abnormalities. *Dermatol Clin* 1985;3:431–43

Daniel CR III, Scher RK. Nail changes secondary to systemic drugs and ingestants. In Daniel CR III, Scher RK, eds. *Nails: Therapy, Diagnosis and Surgery*. Philadelphia: WB Saunders, 1997:251–60

Lateu N, Josette A. Melanonychia: diagnosis and treatment. *Dermatol Ther* 2002;15:131–41

5

Infectious causes of nail disorders

Infections of the nail can be caused by bacteria, virus, fungus and yeast. Fungal infections are the most common infectious process in the nail. Nail infections can be primary or secondary.

Fungal infections of the nail are usually caused by the dermatophytes *Trichophyton rubrum* and *Trichophyton mentagrophytes*. Yeast, such as *Candida albicans*, can infect the nail as a primary or secondary pathogen. Chronic mucocutaneous candidiasis is a rare condition in which *Candida* nail infections occur; however, the secondary appearance of yeast in the nail is the more common presentation. Nails with onycholysis and paronychia are often secondarily infected with *Candida* organism.

ONYCHOMYCOSIS

Onychomycosis is an infection of the nail caused by dermatophytes, yeasts or moulds (Table 3). *Tinea unguium* refers to infection of the nail caused by a dermatophyte. Because the nail can only respond to disease in a limited number of ways, many nail conditions look alike. About 50% of nail diseases are not fungal, so a proper diagnosis is crucial prior to beginning antifungal therapy.

Dermatophytes are fungi that can easily attack the skin, hair and nails due to their keratinolytic enzymes. The prevalence of onychomycosis is in the range of 10–40% of the population, increasing with advancing age. Predisposing factors are a familial history of onychomycosis, diabetes mellitus, immunosuppression and trauma to the nails. Exacerbating factors are excessive perspiration, poorly fitted footwear, and damp feet.

Primary dermatophyte infections occur in four main patterns (Figure 80 and Table 4), as first described by Zaias in 1992.

Distal (and lateral) subungual onychomycosis (Figure 81) is the most common pattern in which

Table 3 Some of the principal organisms found in onychomycosis. Reproduced with permission from Lawry M, Rich P. *Current Problems in Dermatology* 1999;11:161–208

Dermatophytes
  Trichophyton rubrum
  Trichophyton mentagrophytes
  Other dermatophytes occasionally

Yeasts
  Candida albicans and possibly other species

Non-dermatophytes
  Scytalidium dimidiatum
  Scytalidium hyalinum
  Scopulariopsis
  Fusarium species
  Aspergillus species
  Acremonium
  Others

Table 4 Classes of onychomycosis

Distal/lateral subungual onychomycosis

Superficial white onychomycosis

Proximal subungual onychomycosis

Total dystrophic onychomycosis

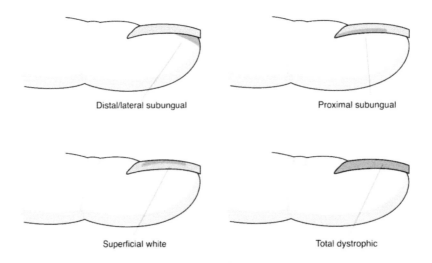

Figure 80   The four main patterns of dermatophyte onychomycosis

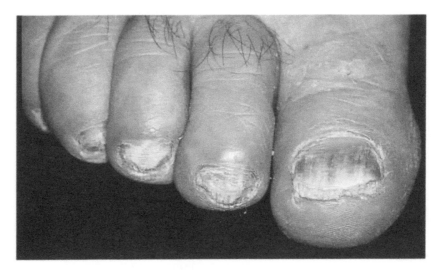

Figure 81   Distal subungual onychomycosis

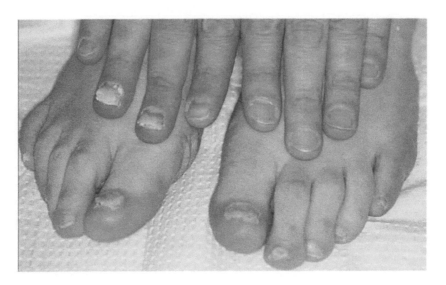

Figure 82   Two-foot one-hand onychomycosis

the nail plate is invaded from the hyponychium. Often, there is concomitant tinea pedis or tinea manum, which may present as two-feet one-hand onychomycosis (Figure 82). The fungus, usually *T. rubrum*, penetrates the nail bed and nail plate from the hyponychium distally. As the process progresses, the nail bed becomes hyperkeratotic (Figure 83). There may be linear yellow streaks (Figure 84) progressing back toward the matrix, which repre-sents the localized focus of fungal organisms. Lateral fungal nail involvement (Figure 85) and yellow longitudinal spikes are associated with a higher risk of treatment failure. There is evidence for a genetic predisposition for *T. rubrum* skin and nail infections.

White superficial onychomycosis (Figure 86) is seen primarily on the toes. The surface of the nail plate is invaded by the fungal organisms and appears white, powdery and sometimes friable. The usual organism

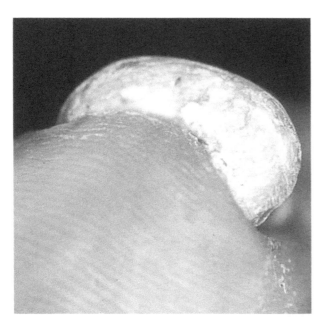

Figure 83   Distal subungual onychomycosis with hyperk-eratosis

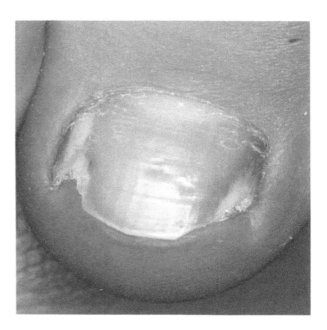

Figure 85   Lateral fungal nail involvement in onychomy-cosis

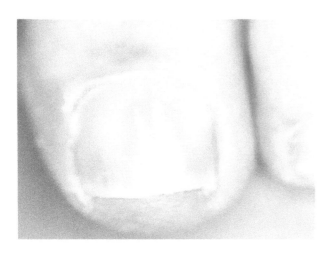

Figure 84   Yellow streaks in onychomycosis, indicating localized foci of fungal organisms

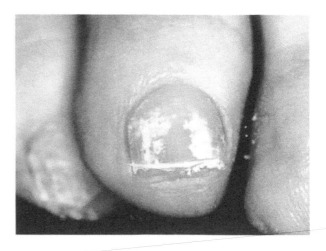

Figure 86   White superficial onychomycosis

involved in white superficial onychomycosis is *T. mentagrophytes*.

Proximal subungual onychomycosis is the least common dermatophyte pattern in the nail and affects the inferior portion of the proximal nail plate. It is believed that the organism gains access to the nail by penetrating the nail cuticle and proximal nail fold and affects the proximal nail plate (Figure 87). The infection spreads in the nail bed in a proximal to distal direction. The usual cause of proximal subun-

gual onychomycosis is *T. rubrum*, but, occasionally, it is caused by some non-dermatophyte moulds. A subtype, called proximal white subungual onychomycosis, is seen in patients with acquired immunodeficiency syndrome and can be the presenting sign of human immunodeficiency virus (HIV) infection.

Total dystrophic onychomycosis (Figure 88) is the result of unchecked progression of any of the three forms of onychomycosis with nail matrix involve-

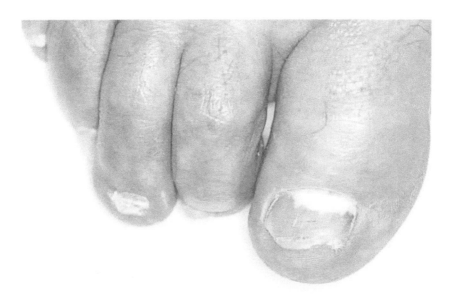

Figure 87   Proximal subungual onychomycosis

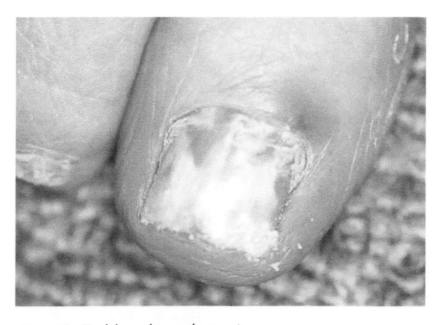

Figure 88   Total dystrophic onychomycosis

ment, although the most common is distal subungual onychomycosis. The nail is usually hyperkeratotic and crumbling.

True *Candida* onychomycosis is rare and occurs primarily in patients who are immunosuppressed, as in chronic mucocandidiasis (Figure 89). *Candida* is not an efficient invader of nail keratin under normal conditions. *Candida* occurs as a secondary infection in onycholysis and paronychia. *Candida albicans* can cause total dystrophic onychomycosis in patients with chronic mucocutaneous candidiasis.

Diagnosis of onychomycosis

Table 5 lists the main methods of diagnosis of onychomycosis. Mycological confirmation of the presence of the causative organism should be performed prior to treatment with an oral antifungal drug. The simplest and quickest method is by using a potassium hydroxide preparation, where the diseased nail plate is clipped and the exposed and diseased debris from the nail bed is scraped and viewed microscopically after the potassium hydroxide digestion (Figure 90). When identification of the

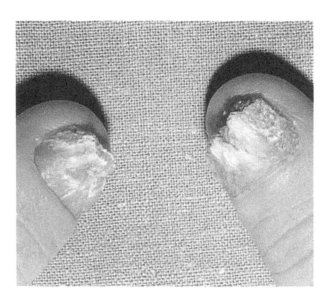

Figure 89 Chronic mucocutaneous candidiasis (courtesy of Jon Hanifin)

Table 5 Diagnosis of onychomycosis

Potassium hydroxide (KOH) preparation of subungual debris
        chlorazole black E
        calciflor white

Culture of nail bed or nail plate debris
        Mycosel, Sabouraud's, dermatophyte test medium

Histology of nail plate and/or nail bed
        periodic acid Schiff (PAS)

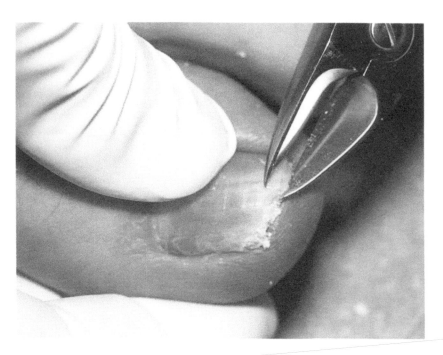

Figure 90 Subungual debris is collected for potassium hydroxide (KOH) examination for the appearance of fungal hyphae

organism is required, a culture of subungual debris can be inoculated on Mycosel and Sabouraud's media (Figure 91).

Treatment of onychomycosis

The treatment of onychomycosis has advanced enormously in the past decade (Table 6). There are several oral antifungal drugs that can be used with high success rates. In the past, griseofulvin and ketoconazole (Nizoral) were used but they both have significant limitations. Griseofulvin is fungistatic and needs to be taken in relatively high doses for 1 year or more for toenails. Ketoconazole use is limited by the potential for hepatotoxicity. Three new drugs have greatly supplemented these older medications. Terbinafine is an allylamine and is prescribed at a dose of 250 mg daily for 12 weeks for toenails and 6 weeks for fingernails. Itraconazole can be given as a continuous dose of 100 mg twice daily for 12 weeks or a pulse dose of 200 mg twice daily for 1 week each month for 3 months. Fluconazole is a triazole with usefulness against yeast and dermatophytes. It is given at a dose of 200 mg once weekly until the nails are normal, a period of time which could be up to 12 months for toenails and 9 months for fingernails. Fluconazole is not approved by the Food and Drug Administration (FDA) for the indication of onychomycosis.

Topical onychomycosis therapy is advancing rapidly. There is one topical antifungal drug, cyclopirox, approved by the FDA for the treatment of onychomycosis, and there are several other topical antifungal drugs in clinical trials for onychomycosis.

Several regimens have been proposed for the use of topical antifungal therapy to keep nails free of fungus after the nails are clear.

BACTERIAL INFECTIONS

Bacteria can invade a weakened or damaged nail. The organism usually gains access through cuts in the nail folds or hyponychium, as in paronychia and onycholysis (Figures 92 and 93). The most common bacterial infection is *Staphylococcus*, which causes an acute red and painful infection. Acute paronychia may cause a pus-filled abscess and should be treated by incision and drainage and a culture-specific antibacterial antibiotic. *Streptococcus* is a less frequent invader of the perionychium and occurs in blistering distal dactylitis (Figure 94), in which there is a nontender blister on the tip of the digit. This condition is usually seen in children and β-hemolytic

Table 6 Current treatment for onychomycosis of fingernails and toenails in adults

---

Topical medications
Cyclopirox lacquer
Other topical antifungal medication in trials

Surgical mechanical removal of nails
Nail avulsion is occasionally helpful for an isolated fungal
  nail resistant to medical therapy
Chemical avulsion using urea paste

Medical therapy (oral)
Older medications for onychomycosis treatment
  Griseofulvin micro 500 bid for as long as it takes for
    the nail to regrow (approximately 12 months for
    toenails)
  Ketoconazole not used due to high risk for
    hepatotoxicity with prolonged treatment course

Current antifungal medications
  Itraconazole
    continuous dosing 100 mg bid for 90 days
    pulse dosing 200 mg bid for 1 week per month × 3
  Terbinafine continuous dosing 250 mg bid for 90 days
  Fluconazole 200 mg p.o. weekly until nails are clear
    (not approved by the FDA for the indication of
    onychomycosis)

Combination treatment
Surgical removal with oral or topical antifungal used
  during regrowth

Medical therapy that combines topical and oral therapy

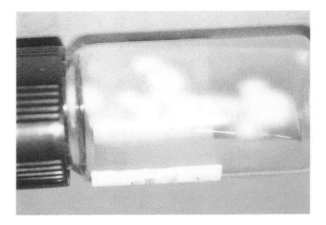

Figure 91 Culture for identification of fungus

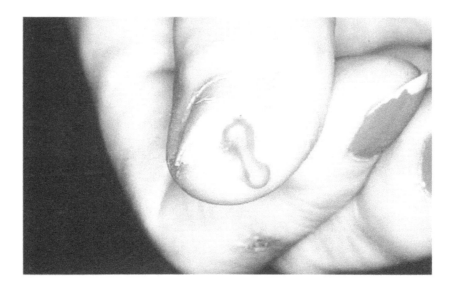

Figure 92 Acute bacterial paronychia

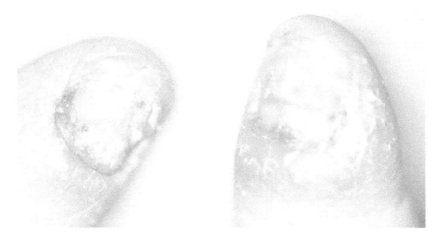

Figure 93 *Candida* onychomycosis and paronychia in a child who sucks his fingers, with secondary bacterial infection

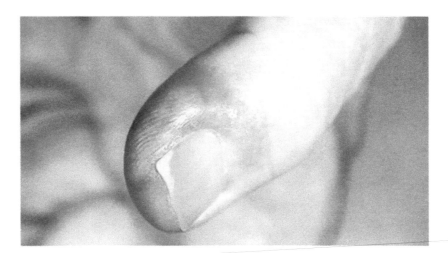

Figure 94 Blistering distal dactylitis is due to *Streptococcus* and occurs in the fingertips in children

streptococcus can be cultured from the blister fluid (see acute paronychia).

Pseudomonas is a water-borne bacterium that may secondarily affect a damaged or injured nail (Figure 95). It is often seen in onycholysis and may also affect psoriatic nails. The organism is easily treated by dilute acetic acid (vinegar) or gentamycin solution but the blue–green pigment, a pyocyanin, may persist.

VIRAL INFECTIONS

The most common viral infection of the nail is verruca vulgaris, caused by the human papillomavirus (Figures 96 and 97). Periungual and subungual warts can be particularly resistant to treatment, and over-zealous treatment in the area of the nail matrix can result in permanent nail dystrophy. Warts that persist after treatment should be biopsied to rule out squamous cell carcinoma *in situ*, which can mimic warts (Figure 98).

Herpetic whitlow can occur around the nails in dentists and others exposed to active herpes simplex virus lesions (Figure 99).

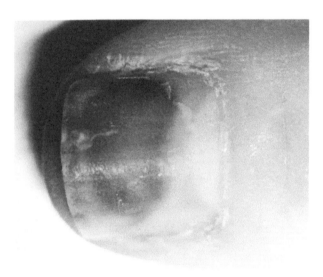

Figure 95 Secondary involvement by *Pseudomonas* in an onycholytic nail

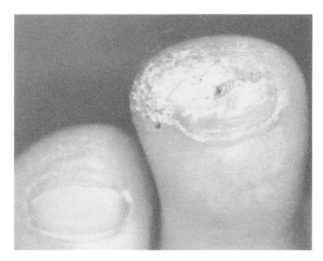

Figure 97 Periungual wart on toe

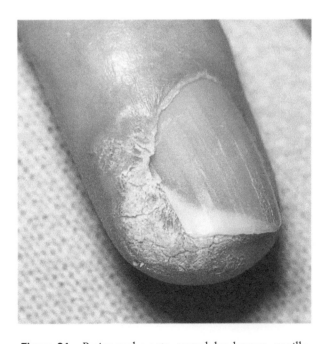

Figure 96 Periungual warts caused by human papillomavirus

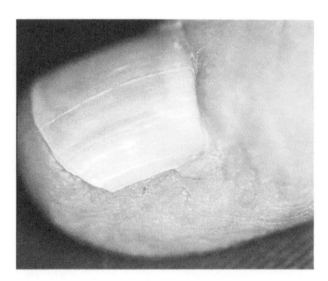

Figure 98 Bowen's disease of the proximal and lateral nail fold mimicking a wart present for 23 years

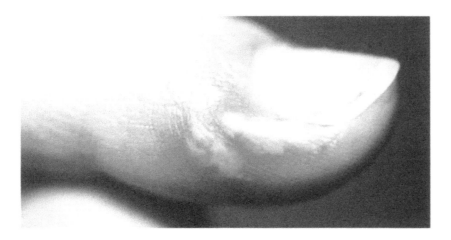

Figure 99 Herpetic whitlow

FURTHER READING

Daniel CR III, Scher RK. Nail changes secondary to systemic drugs and ingestants. In Daniel CR III, Scher RK, eds. *Nails: Therapy, Diagnosis, and Surgery*, 2nd edn. Philadelphia: WB Saunders, 1997:251–60

Elewski BE, Charif M, Daniel CR. Onychomycosis. In Scher RK, Daniel CR III, eds. *Nails: Therapy, Diagnosis and Management*, 2nd edn. Philadelphia: WB Saunders, 1997:151–61

Fleckman P. Onychomycosis: diagnosis and topical therapy. *Dermatol Ther* 2002;15:

Hay RJ, Baran R, Haneke E. Fungal and other infections of the nail apparatus. In Baran R, Dawber RPR, eds. *Diseases of the Nails and Their Management*, 3rd edn. Oxford: Blackwell Scientific, 2001:129–41

Hay RJ, Baran R, Moore MK, Wilkinson JD. Candida onychomycosis – and evaluation of the role of Candida species in nail disease. *Br J Dermatol* 1988;118:47–58

Rebell G, Zaias N. Introducing the syndromes of human dermatophytosis. *Cutis* 2001;67:6–17

Tosti A, Piraccini BM, Ghetti E, Colombo MD. Topical steroids versus systemic antifungals in the treatment of chronic paronychia: an open, randomized double-blind and double dummy study. *J Am Acad Dermatol* 2002;47:73–6

Wollina U. Acute paronychia: comparative treatment with topical antibiotic alone or in combination with corticosteroid. *J Eur Acad Dermatol Venereol* 2001;15:82–4

Zaias N. *The Nail in Health and Disease*, 2nd edn. Norwalk, CT: Appleton and Lange, 1990:1–255

6

Nail manifestations of cutaneous disease

PSORIASIS

Psoriasis is a cutaneous disorder that causes increased cell proliferation and affects skin and nails. Nail psoriasis is the most common nail disorder that is associated with cutaneous disease. Psoriasis of the nails occurs in more that 50% of people with cutaneous psoriasis. Psoriasis limited to the nails is seen in about 5% of psoriatics and sometimes presents a diagnostic challenge. Minimal changes of the scalp, umbilicus or gluteal cleft can sometimes be found and confirm the diagnosis. When psoriatic arthritis of the fingers is present, there is an 86% chance of finding psoriasis in the nails. The clinical features of psoriasis of the nails depend upon which part of the nail unit is involved (Table 7 and Figure 100).

Table 7 The clinical features of nail psoriasis are dependent on the location in the nail unit

Location	Features
Nail matrix	pitting
	leukonychia
	red spots in lunula
Nail bed	'oil drop' (salmon patches)
	nail bed hyperkeratosis
	splinter hemorrhages
Proximal nail fold	cutaneous psoriasis
Hyponychium	hyperkeratosis

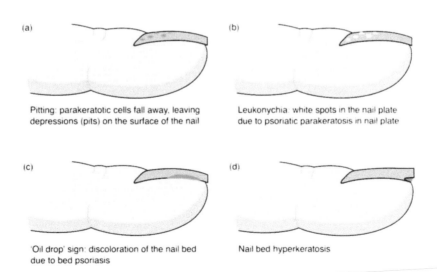

(a) Pitting: parakeratotic cells fall away, leaving depressions (pits) on the surface of the nail

(b) Leukonychia: white spots in the nail plate due to psoriatic parakeratosis in nail plate

(c) 'Oil drop' sign: discoloration of the nail bed due to bed psoriasis

(d) Nail bed hyperkeratosis

Figure 100 Diagram showing how nail matrix and nail bed psoriasis result in clinical features of psoriasis

Pitting (Figure 101) is the most common sign of nail psoriasis and indicates nail matrix involvement. There may be small pits or large transverse furrows, indicating longer duration of psoriasis in the matrix (Figures 102 and 103). Pitting occurs when small foci of parakeratotic cells occur in the nail plate and then fall out after the nail pit grows past the cuticle, leaving a depression in the nail plate (Figure 104). Other signs of nail psoriasis are 'oil-drop' discoloration (Figure 105) or salmon-colored areas of varying size in the nail. These are due to nail bed and, sometimes, distal nail matrix psoriasis. As the nail grows, the 'oil drop' moves distally and eventually becomes nail bed hyperkeratosis (Figure 106)

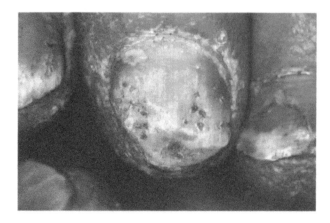

Figure 103 Leukonychia and pitting due to psoriasis in the nail matrix

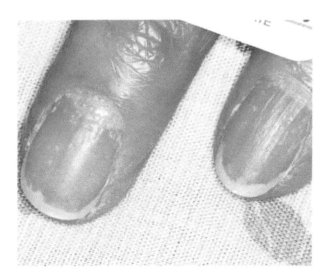

Figure 101 Pitting is a common sign of nail psoriasis

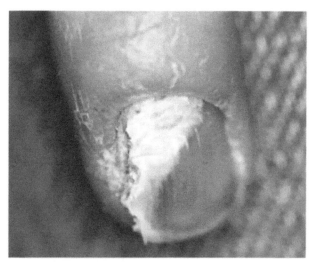

Figure 104 Pitting due to psoriasis, showing a depression in the nail plate (Beau's lines)

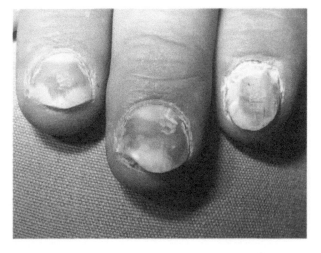

Figure 102 Pitting indicating a longer duration of psoriasis in the matrix

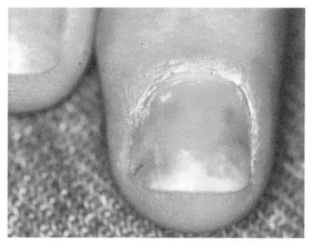

Figure 105 'Oil-drop' discoloration in psoriasis

and onycholysis. Psoriatic onycholysis (Figure 107), splinter hemorrhages (Figure 108), and hyperkeratosis are the result of psoriasis in the nail bed and hyponychium. Psoriasis of the proximal nail fold resembles psoriasis in skin and is sometimes associated with chronic paronychia and nail plate irregularities (Figure 109). Nail psoriasis can be easily confused with onychomycosis. Chronic paronychia can sometimes be associated with nail psoriasis. The isomorphic phenomenon or Koebner reaction can occur in the nail unit, resulting in exacerbation of nail psoriasis following minor trauma to the nail. Psoriasis of the nails is generally self-limiting and will not result in scarring.

The diagnosis of nail psoriasis is usually made by clinical features and the presence of cutaneous psoriasis elsewhere. KOH wet mount examination should be performed because clinical presentation can be identical to dermatophytic infections. Psoriasis of the nail occurs in up to 40% of children with psoriasis. It can have typical psoriatic nail findings or present as trachyonychia (Figure 110). Parakeratosis

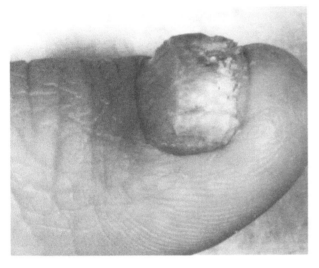

Figure 106 Nail bed hyperkeratosis in psoriatic nail

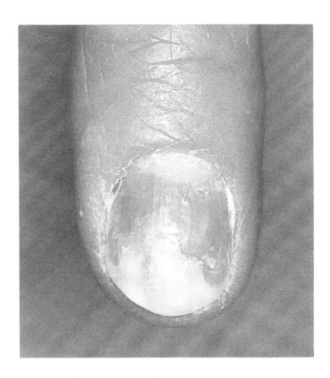

Figure 107 Psoriatic onycholysis

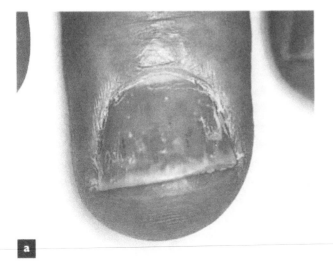

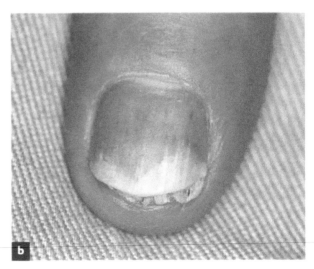

Figure 108 Splinter hemorrhages in psoriasis

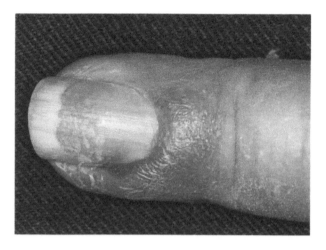

Figure 109 Psoriasis of the proximal nail fold, showing chronic paronychia and nail plate irregularities

pustulosa (Figures 111 and 112) is a self-limiting form of nail psoriasis that usually affects young girls; it spontaneously resolves (*see* Chapter 8).

The nail changes seen in Reiter's syndrome are similar to those seen in psoriasis, with the added feature of paronychial scaling and inflammation (Figure 113). Pustular psoriasis of the nails can progress rapidly and result in scarring of the nails. Oral retinoid therapy is often used in patients with severe pustular psoriasis involving the nails (Figure 114).

Treatment

Treatment of nail psoriasis needs patience and motivation on behalf of the patient. It takes many months

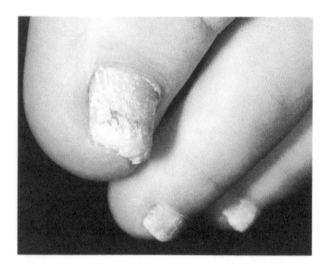

Figure 110 Trachyonychia in a child with psoriasis

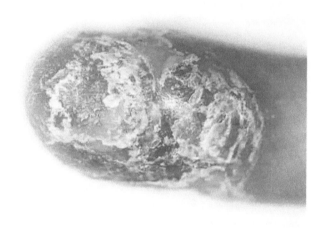

Figure 111 Pustular psoriasis

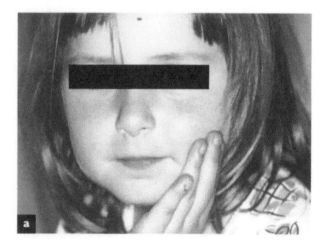

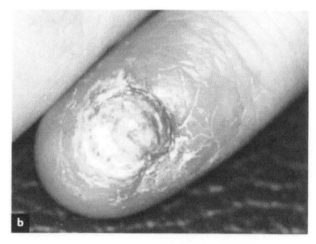

Figure 112 (a) Parakeratosis pustulosa in a young girl. A close-up view of the nail is shown in (b)

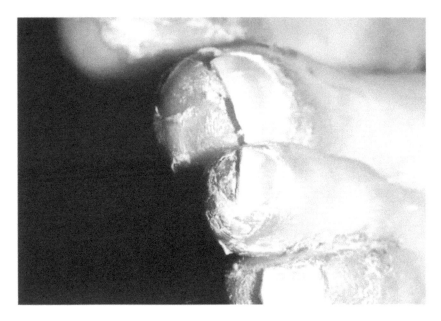

Figure 113 Nail changes in a patient with Reiter's syndrome, showing parony-chial scaling and inflammation

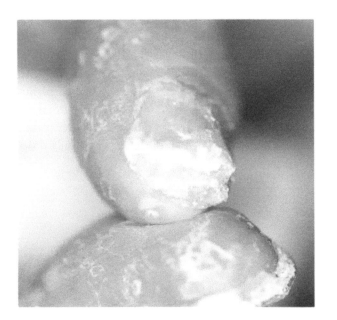

Figure 114 Pustular psoriasis involving the nails

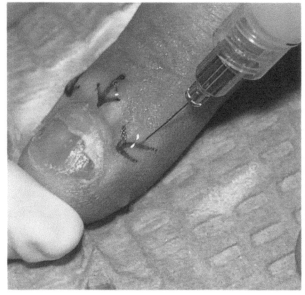

Figure 115 Intralesional injections of cortisone into the proximal nail fold for psoriasis

to see results and the nails are subject to relapse. Topical therapy consists of high-potency cortico-steroids applied around and under the nail with or without occlusion. Topical calcipotriol and tazaro-tene can be tried. The most effective treatment for nail psoriasis is intralesional cortisone injection of triamcinolone acetonide into the proximal nail fold

for pitting due to matrix involvement (Figure 115). With nail bed involvement, the intralesional injec-tions are performed in the lateral nail fold so that the drug diffuses into the nail bed. The usual dose is 2.5–3 mg/ml diluted with plain lidocaine and injected with a 30-gauge needle after the nail fold is sprayed with a coolant to reduce discomfort.

Occasionally, a subungual hemorrhage will occur following injection (Figure 116). Systemic treatments such as PUVA (psoralen plus ultraviolet light of the A wavelength), methotrexate, cyclosporin, or etretinate are sometimes used, but these drugs are usually reserved for extensive cutaneous psoriasis rather than for psoriasis limited to the nails. Psoriasis

can be exacerbated by some medications, such as lithium and β-blockers, and *Streptococcal* infections. Up to 80% of patients with psoriatic arthritis of the distal interphalangeal joints have nail psoriasis (Figure 117).

LICHEN PLANUS

Nail involvement occurs in about 10% of patients with lichen planus, a condition of unknown etiology. Approximately 25% of patients with lichen planus of the nails have lichen planus in other sites of the skin, hair or mucous membranes, before or after the nail lesions appear. The clinical features of lichen planus depend upon which portion of the nail unit is affected. Lichen planus can cause longitudinal ridging (Figure 118) of the nail plate, with eventual nail plate thinning. With advanced disease, there can be scarring of the matrix that causes pterygium (a wing-like permanent nail dystrophy) (Figure 119) and anonychia (Figure 120). Occasionally, lichen planus of the nail can be ulcerative (Figure 121). A nail matrix biopsy of suspected lichen planus shows typical lichenoid infiltrate. Because permanent nail dystrophy may be seen in up to 40% of patients with nail lichen planus, rapidly progressive lichen planus should be treated aggressively to prevent permanent loss of the nails. Rapidly destructive lichen planus should be treated with oral prednisone at daily doses

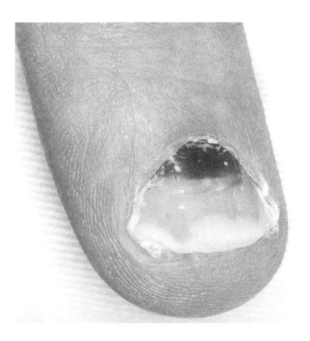

Figure 116 Subungual hemorrhage following intralesional injection for psoriasis

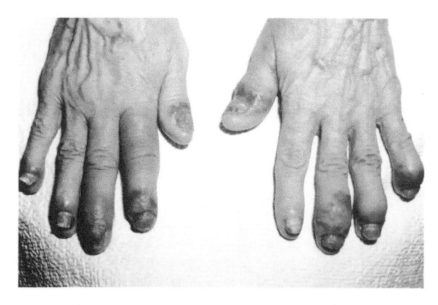

Figure 117 Nail psoriasis is common in psoriatic arthritis of the distal interphalangeal joints. (Photo courtesy of Oregon Dermatology Department)

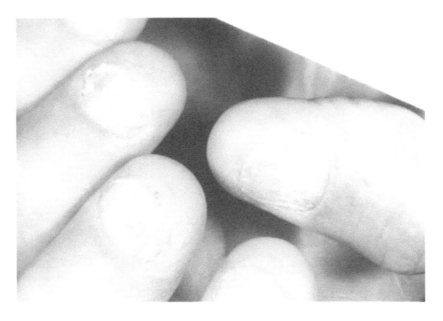

Figure 118 Longitudinal ridging (onychorrhexis) in lichen planus

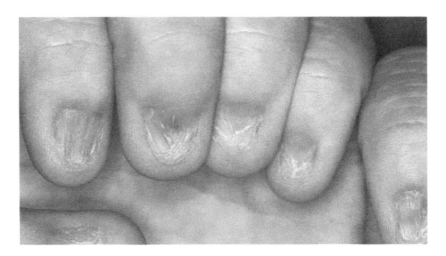

Figure 119 Pterygium in advanced lichen planus

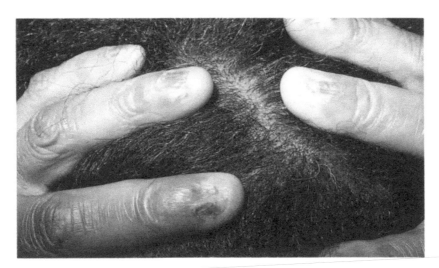

Figure 120 Anonychia in advanced lichen planus associated with lichen plano-pilaris of the scalp

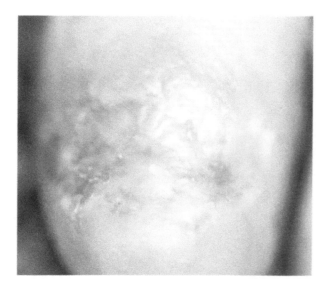

Figure 121 Ulcerative lichen planus of the nail

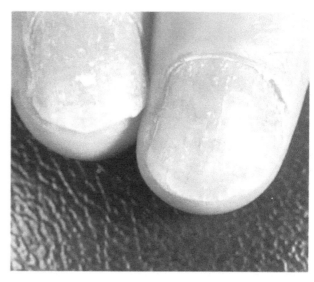

Figure 122 Pitting of the nail in alopecia areata

of 40–60 mg, decreasing over 4–6 weeks, intralesional triamcinolone 2.5 mg into the proximal nail fold or intramuscular triamcinolone. Lichen planus occurs in adults and children and, if the diagnosis is in question, a biopsy of the nail matrix is usually conclusive.

ALOPECIA AREATA

Alopecia areata is a condition that causes both hair loss and nail changes, although not necessarily at the same time. Nail changes caused by alopecia areata are pitting (Figure 122), thinning of the nail plate (Figure 123) and sometimes red lunula (Figure 124). Topical and intralesional triamcinolone 2.5–3 mg/ml at monthly intervals are helpful when spontaneous clearing of the nails does not occur. Pitting, trachyonychia (rough sandpapered surface), Beau's lines and onychomadesis can be seen in nail alopecia areata. Pink spots in the lunula are often seen in alopecia areata of the nails (Figure 123). Nail changes in alopecia areata are more common in children, with more than 46% of 272 children with alopecia areata having nail involvement. In adults, nail changes occur in about one-fifth of patients who present with alopecia areata of the scalp.

If the diagnosis of alopecia areata is not readily apparent, a biopsy of the nail matrix shows spongiosis, which is distinguished from eczematous nail changes by the absence of dermatitis of the paronychial folds.

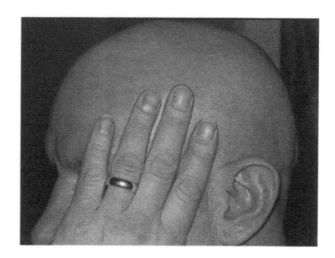

Figure 123 Alopecia areata of the nails, showing thinning of the nail plate

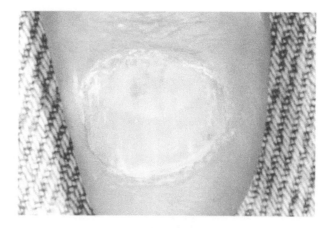

Figure 124 The red spot in the lunula

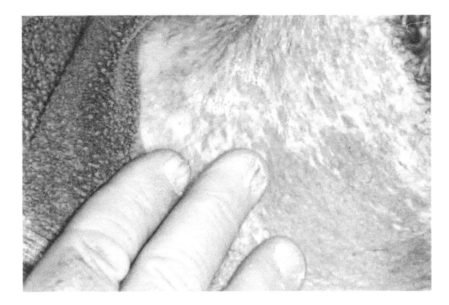

Figure 125 Nail changes in Darier's disease

DARIER'S DISEASE

Darier's disease, also known as keratosis follicularis, is an autosomal dominantly inherited condition with nail involvement in 90% of patients. Involvement of the nail matrix results in onychorrhexis, with splitting and fragility as well as red and white longitudinal streaks. When Darier's disease affects the distal nail bed, there is subungual hyperkeratosis, with overlying V-shaped notches at the free edge (Figure 125).

FURTHER READING

Farber EM, Nall L. Nail psoriasis. *Cutis* 1992;50:174

Jones SM, Armas JB, Cohen MG, *et al.* Psoriatic arthritis: disease subsets and relationshops of joint disease to nail and skin disease. *Br J Rheumatol* 1994;33:834

Scher RK. Psoriasis of the nail. *Dermatol Clin* 1985;3:387

Zaias N. Psoriasis of the nail: a clinico-pathological study. *Arch Dermatol* 1969;99:567–79

7

Nail signs of systemic disease

Nail changes can be a clue to systemic disease. Many nail signs are specific for certain internal diseases and many more are not specific but still valuable clues that further work-up for internal disease is warranted. Many of the nail signs are reaction patterns that can be associated with multiple organ system disorders. Some of the more common nail signs will be discussed as they relate to organ systems and systemic disease.

KOILONYCHIA

Koilonychia, commonly called spoon nails, occurs when the free edge of the nail is everted (Figure 126). Koilonychia can be idiopathic or associated with a variety of conditions such as anemia, occupational and traumatic injury, or endocrine conditions such as hypo- and hyperthyroidism. Koilonychia is a common occurrence in the healthy toenails of young children.

DIGITAL CLUBBING

Digital clubbing has been on the minds of clinicians since the days of Hippocrates. Clubbing is characterized by increases in distal finger tip mass and increased longitudinal and horizontal curvature of the nail plate (Figure 127). Clubbing affects the fingernails and toenails (Figure 128). Stone and

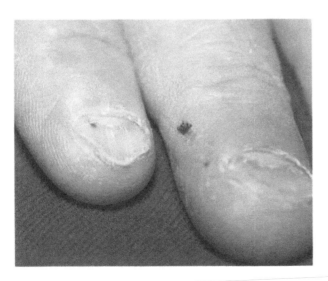

Figure 126 Koilonychia, or spoon nails, showing the everted free edges of the nails

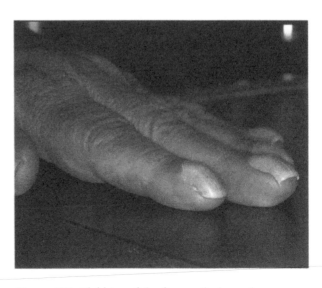

Figure 127 Clubbing of the fingernails due to lung cancer

colleagues classified clubbing into three convenient categories: congenital/hereditary, acquired and idiopathic. Clinical findings of clubbing are the abnormal curvature of the nail plate in both the longitudinal and horizontal axes. In clubbing, the angle of Lovibond (the angle between the nail plate and the proximal nail fold when viewed from the side) is greater than 180°, whereas, in normal nails, the angle is less than 160°. There is also bulbous enlargement of the pulp of the distal digit (Figure 129). While advanced clubbing is easy to recognize, early clubbing is quite subtle.

Acquired clubbing is the most important category. Most of the time, clubbing means that something is not going well for the body. Infectious, neoplastic and inflammatory pulmonary problems are most common. Pulmonary problems such as neoplasms of the lung, bronchiectasis, emphysema, pneumonia and lymphoma are all possible.

Cardiovascular etiologies such as congestive heart failure, and congenital heart/valve disease pertain, as do gastrointestinal and hepatic disorders such as cirrhosis and ulcerative colitis. Idiopathic and congenital categories are less common.

BEAU'S LINES

Beau's lines are transverse depressions in one or more nails that result from a growth arrest in the nail matrix following a systemic illness or severe trauma. These grooves grow out with the nail, and, because nails grow at a constant rate, the time of the insult can be calculated. Beau's lines can be narrow or

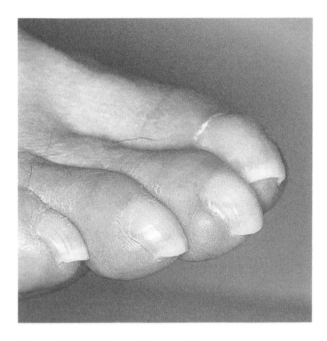

Figure 128 Clubbing of the toenails

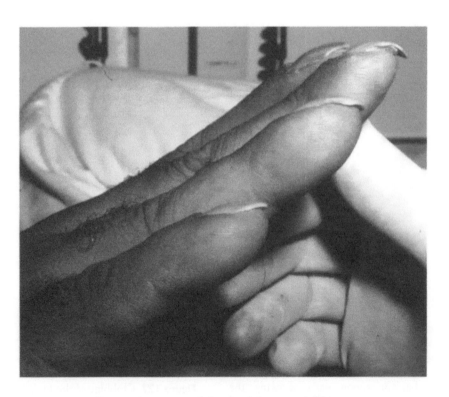

Figure 129 Bulbous enlargement of the distal digits in clubbing

wide, indicating the duration of the systemic insult (Figure 130).

HALF-AND-HALF NAILS

Half-and-half nails are described as having a proximal white half and a distal red/brown half due to changes in the nail bed color. Half-and-half nails occur as a sign of renal insufficiency and uremia. The nails revert to normal when renal function normalizes or following renal transplant (Figure 131).

TERRY'S NAILS

Terry's nails are described as milky white nails that extend from the proximal nail fold to the narrow red–brown band in the area of the onychodermal band on the nail. The lunula is usually obscured by the white. Pressing on the nail plate alters the

appearance and color of the nail. Terry's nails have been associated with congestive heart failure, liver disease and even aging (Figure 132).

RED LUNULAS

Red lunulas are a non-specific finding in such disparate conditions as rheumatoid arthritis, alopecia areata, congestive heart failure, pulmonary disorders and carbon monoxide poisoning. The pathogenic mechanism of the erythema of the lunula is unknown.

SPLINTER HEMORRHAGES

Splinter hemorrhages (Figure 133) are a non-specific nail change characterized by small linear dark

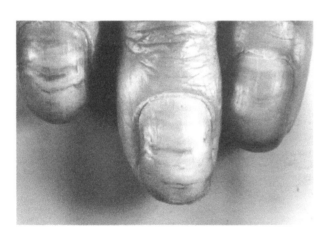

Figure 130 Beau's lines

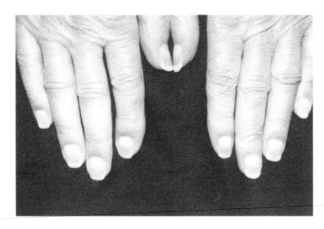

Figure 131 Half-and-half nails

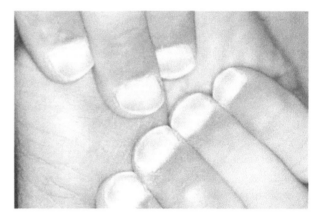

Figure 132 Terry's nails

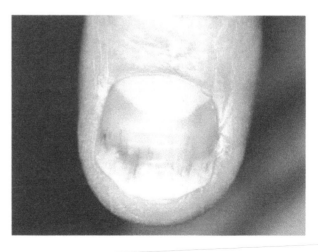

Figure 133 Splinter hemorrhages are linear dark streaks in the nail bed and are associated with trauma, psoriasis and, less commonly, endocarditis and trichinosis

red/brown lines in the nail bed that are oriented in the longitudinal axis. They are asymptomatic and usually occur in the distal portion of the nail. They are the result of tiny amounts of blood in the longitudinal grooves of the nail bed. The most common cause of splinter hemorrhage is trauma. Some psoriatic nails exhibit splinter hemorrhages resulting from tiny nail bed microhemorrhages. There is a long list of less common conditions in which splinter hemorrhages are found including trichinosis, endocarditis, embolic events, blood dyscrasias, and with certain medications.

CONNECTIVE TISSUE AND SOME RHEUMATOLOGIC DISORDERS

Clues to the diagnosis of some collagen vascular diseases can be obtained by visualization of the capillaries in the proximal nail folds. Some connective tissue disorders have abnormalities of the size and spacing of the capillaries of the proximal nail fold. With capillary microscopy, the vessels can be visualized by placing a drop of mineral oil on the nail fold and viewing with magnification such as an ophthalmoscope. The vascular supply of the normal proximal nail fold has regular spacing of capillaries, which are of uniform size and density. In scleroderma and dermatomyositis, there are fewer capillaries present, many of which have enlarged dilated loops. Systemic lupus also has dilated capillaries but there are no skip or avascular areas.

Scleroderma

Systemic sclerosis produces tapered fingers with avascualar periungual ischemia and may produce

painful keratotic ulcerations in the finger tips due to ischemia. The nail fold capillaries show avascular areas and dilated capillary loops. There may also be inverse pterygium (Figures 134 and 135).

Dermatomyositis

The salient nail findings in dermatomyositis are nail fold erythema and abnormal telangiectasia. There may be hemorrhages in the cuticles which may be thickened (Figure 136).

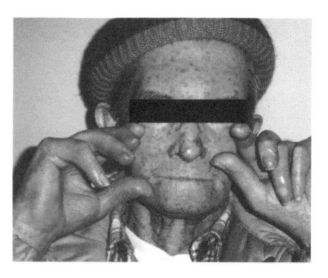

Figure 135 Sclerodactyly and telangiectasis in a patient with CREST syndrome (courtesy of Oregon Dermatology Department)

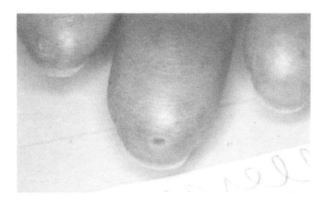

Figure 134 Scleroderma inverse pterygium

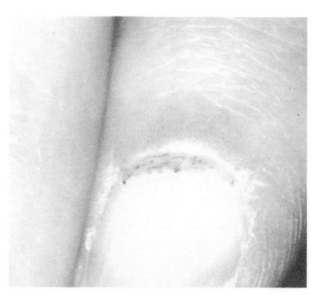

Figure 136 Dermatomyositis: small hemorrhages in cuticle

Systemic lupus erythematosus

The ischemic features of systemic lupus erythematosus (SLE) cause the majority of the nail changes, which are highly variable in presentation. Vascular infarction, nail fold micronecrosis and cuticular vascular lesions are fairly common. In more severe cases, there may be severe necrosis and gangrene due to vascular thrombosis in vessels of the extremity (Figures 137 and 138).

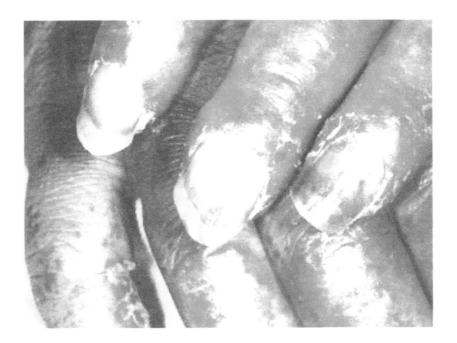

Figure 137 Systemic lupus erythematosus

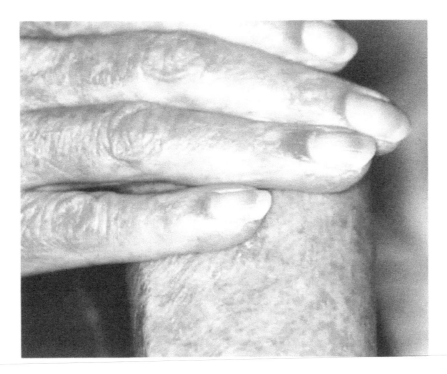

Figure 138 Dilated nail fold capillaries in a patient with systemic lupus erythematosus

Raynaud's syndrome

Chronic Raynaud's syndrome can result in variable nail changes, including thin ridged brittle nails (Figure 139) and, in severe cases, acrosclerosis.

Reiter's disease

The nail changes in patients with Reiter's syndrome are similar to psoriasis and consist of subungual hyperkeratosis, onycholysis, and brownish discoloration. Pitting has been described in some patients (Figure 140).

Pernio

Pernio, or chilblains, is a condition that results from intolerance to cold. The typical lesions are erythematosus, symmetrical itching or burning macules, and papules in the periungual area (Figure 141). Cold avoidance is the usual treatment.

Yellow nail syndrome

Yellow nail syndrome was first described by Samman and White and is characterized by nails that are yellow, slow-growing, with absent lunula and cuticle (Figure 142). The nails may thicken and appear curved and become opaque so that the lunula is obscured, and there may be onycholysis. Conditions associated with yellow nail syndrome are lymphedema, respiratory conditions, including bronchiectasis, sinusitis, and pulmonary effusion. It is sometimes the presenting feature of carcinoma of the lung. There are reports of yellow nail syndrome responding to oral vitamin E therapy.

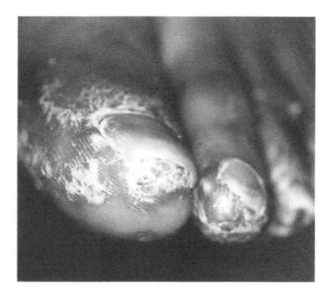

Figure 140 Reiter's disease

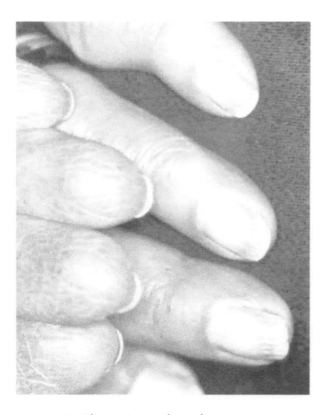

Figure 139 Chronic Raynaud's syndrome

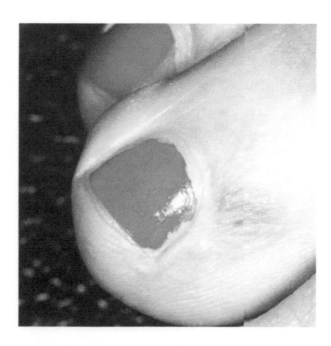

Figure 141 Erythematous tender papules of pernio in periungual area

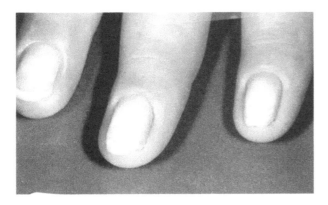

Figure 142 Yellow, thick slow-growing nails in yellow nail syndrome

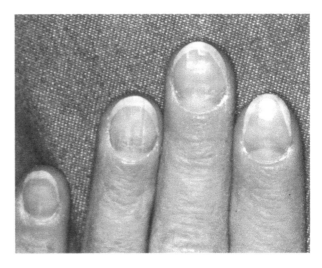

Figure 144 Pigmentation change caused by minocycline

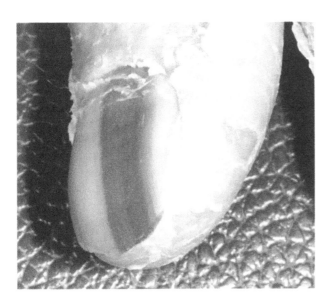

Figure 143 Pigmentation change caused by hydroxyurea

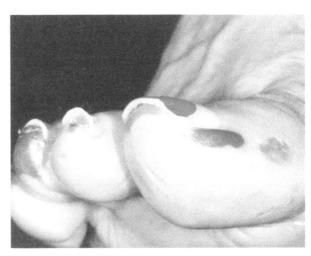

Figure 145 Hemorrhagic bullae in hand-foot syndrome from the medication Xeloda for breast cancer

NAIL CHANGES DUE TO DRUGS

Many medications have the potential to cause changes in the nails such as color changes, nail plate irregularities and abnormalities of the periungual tissue. Antibiotics, retinoids, antineoplastic drugs, and antimalarials are the most likely to cause nail abnormalities. Many changes involve focal or diffuse color change of the nail such as with hydroxyurea (Figure 143) and minocycline (Figure 144). Some drugs cause abnormalities of the nail plate and nail bed, including pitting, onycholysis and splinter hemorrhages or abnormalities of periungual tissue

(Figure 145). There are excellent comprehensive lists of drug effects on the nails that should be used as references.

FURTHER READING

Baran R, Dawber RPR, eds. *Diseases of the Nails and Their Management*, 3rd edn. Oxford: Blackwell Science, 2001

Daniel CR III, Sams WM, Scher RK. Nails in systemic disease. *Dermatol Clin* 1985;3:167–87

Daniel CR III, Sams WM, Scher RK. Nails in systemic disease. In Scher RK, Daniel CR III, eds. *Nails. Therapy,*

Diagnosis and Surgery. Philadelphia: WB Saunders, 1997:219–44

Holzberg M, Walker HK. Terry's nails: revised definition and new correlations. *Lancet* 1984;2:896

Kundu AK. Digital index – a new way of numerical assessment of clubbing. *J Assoc Physicians India* 1999;47:462

Myers KA, Farquhar DR. The rational clinical examination. Does this patient have clubbing? *J Am Med Assoc* 2001;286:341–7

Stone O. Spoon nails and clubbing. *Cutis* 1975;16:235

Vasquez-Abad D, Pineda C, Martinez-Lavin M. Digital clubbing: a numerical assessment of the deformity. *J Rheumatol* 1989;16:518–20

Zaias N. Yellow nail syndrome. In Zaias N, ed. *The Nail in Health and Disease*, 2nd edn. Norwalk CT: Appleton and Lange, 1990: 205–7

8

Age-associated nail disorders

Nail conditions can be lifelong, as in genetic and heredity disorders, or can be present during a particular period of life. While many nail disorders do not discriminate by age, some nail problems have a predilection for geriatric or pediatric patients.

Pediatric nail disorders can be inherited or acquired. Many genodermatoses have nail manifestations that are present at birth or develop early in life.

INHERITED PEDIATRIC NAIL PROBLEMS

Pachyonychia congenita

Pachyonychia congenita is an autosomal dominant inherited condition in which there is massive thickening of the nail bed and brown discoloration of the nail plate (Figures 146–148). In this syndrome, there may be natal teeth and leukokeratosis oris. The molecular basis of pachyonychia congenita is a mutation in keratin 16 and 17[1]. There are four types of pachyonychia congenita with various findings, including follicular and palmar hyperkeratosis, corneal dyskeratosis, cataracts, and dental abnormalities.

Ectodermal dysplasia

Many genodermatoses have skin, hair, teeth and nail manifestations. One example of a genodermatosis that has hair and nail manifestations is hidrotic ectodermal dysplasia (Clouston syndrome)[2]. In this X-linked condition, the hair is sparse, nails are severely

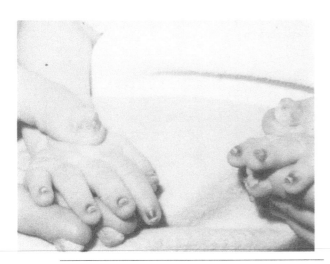

Figure 146 Pachyonychia congenita

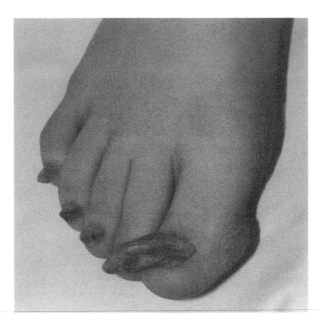

Figure 147 Pachyonychia congenita (courtesy of Ken Lee, MD)

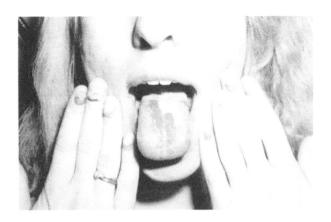

Figure 148 Leukokeratosis oris and nail dystrophy in pachyonychia congenita

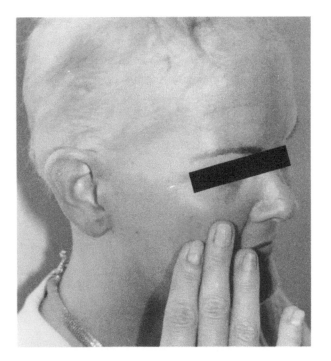

Figure 149 Clouston syndrome

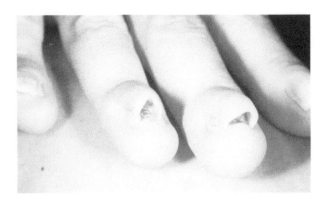

Figure 150 Severely dystrophic nails in Clouston syndrome

dystrophic and there is plantar hyperkeratosis (Figures 149 and 150). Sweating and teeth are normal in this form of ectodermal dysplasia.

When faced with an unusual nail condition suspected of being associated with a genetic syndrome, a good resource database for inherited syndromes is OMIM (Online Mendelian Inheritance in Man). This free website contains an exhaustive database where clinical features can be evaluated in relationship to various genodermatoses.

Epidermolysis bullosa

There are well over 20 different varieties of epidermolysis bullosa, some of which have nail changes. In the autosomal dominant epidermolysis bullosa simplex, the nails may be normal early in life, although repeated traumas usually lead to scarring and dystrophy (Figures 151 and 152). In dystrophic epidermolysis bullosa, there is scarring with mitten-

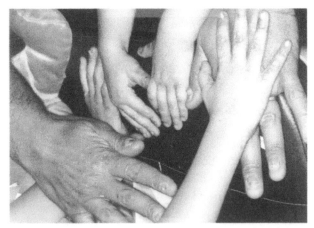

Figure 151 Epidermolysis bullosa simplex in father and two children

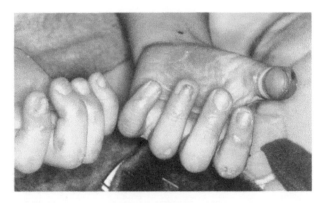

Figure 152 Epidermolysis bullosa simplex nail dystrophy

like deformity of the digits due to loss of matrix from a split in the dermis beneath the matrix. In junctional and acquired epidermolysis bullosa, the nails are thickened and dystrophic.

Nail patella syndrome

Nail patella syndrome, also called osteo-onychodysplasia, is characterized by nails that have triangular or V-shaped lunula. The X-ray finding shows an aplastic patella, resulting in pain with exercise. Many patients with this syndrome have kidney and ocular abnormalities.

Trichothiodystrophy

Patients with trichothiodystrophy present with brittle hair and brittle nails due to a defect in cystine-rich proteins in the matrix. The nails may be thin, split, and spooned.

Linear epidermal nevus

Linear epidermal nevus can affect the nail unit if the nevus runs down the digit and involves the nail matrix. In this situation, the nail fold and nail plate are involved and a linear dystrophy in the nail is present (Figure 153).

Congenital malalignment of the great toenails

Congenital malalignment of the great toenails is characterized by lateral deviation of one or both great toe nails. Often the nails thicken and develop horizontal ridges and discoloration. The condition is present at birth and often runs in families (Figure 154). Rarely does it affect fingernails. An elaborate surgical procedure, that involves rotating the matrix into alignment with the longitudinal axis of the digit, has been employed[3,4].

ACQUIRED PEDIATRIC NAIL PROBLEMS

Beau's lines

Beau's lines are due to a mild growth arrest causing a transverse depression in the nail plate that reflects the timing and duration of the event[5]. Nearly any moderate stress on the system, such as surgery or high fever, can result in their appearance. Beau's lines are sometimes seen 1–2 months after a traumatic delivery (Figure 155).

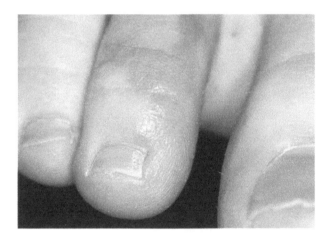

Figure 153 Linear dystrophy in linear epidermal nevus

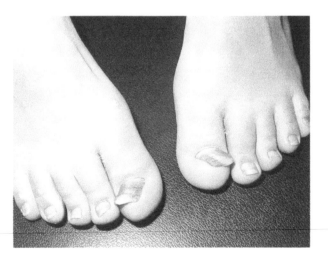

Figure 154 Congenital malalignment of the great toenail

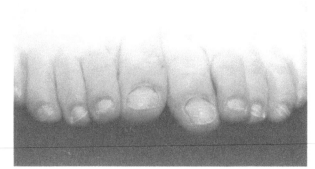

Figure 155 Beau's lines

Onychomadesis

Onychomadesis occurs in the setting of a complete growth arrest that progresses to shedding of the nails. It can occur in fingernails or toenails. It occurs in children in the setting of a severe systemic infection and can also be idiopathic[6-8]. The nails regrow completely and spontaneously without scarring. Viral infections such as hand, foot and mouth disease and drug reactions have been reported to cause onychomadesis in children.

Lichen striatus

Lichen striatus is a linear inflammatory skin condition that results in hyperkeratotic skin changes along the length of an extremity[9]. When it extends to the nail unit and involves the proximal nail fold, there is often an associated longitudinal ridged nail dystrophy. The cause of lichen striatus is unknown and it usually resolves spontaneously over several years (Figure 156).

Eczema

Fifty percent of patients with atopic dermatitis are diagnosed by age 1 year. The clinical distribution of atopic dermatitis in young children is facial and extensor, whereas, in adults, it is more flexural with hand involvement. Hand eczema around the proximal nail fold and the cuticle results in stippling and pitting of the nail due to the disruption of the nail fold. Shiny buffed nails occur in children who have atopic dermatitis and scratch frequently, buffing their nails to a shine. In addition to irritant avoidance, treatment of nail fold eczema is topical corticosteroids and topical immune response modifiers. After the eczema is clear and the cuticle attaches to the nail plate, the nail usually grows in smoothly again.

PEDIATRIC INFECTIONS OF THE NAIL UNIT

Bacterial, fungal and viral infections occur in the pediatric population as well as in adults.

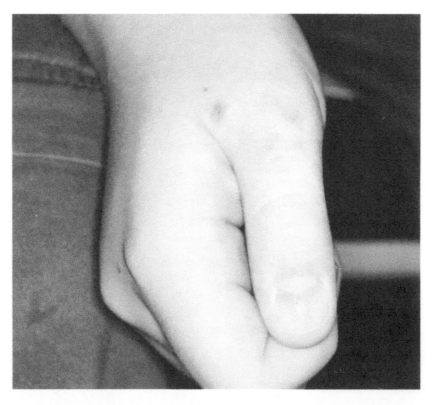

Figure 156 Lichen striatus causes a linear nail dystrophy when it extends from the dorsum of the digit to the proximal nail fold

Viral infections

The most common viral infections in children are viral warts and herpes simplex whitlow. Verruca vulgaris (common warts) in a periungual distribution is very common in children and adolescents. Human papillomavirus in the periungual location are types 1, 2 and 4 and are most common around the nails. Warts can access to the skin through small abrasions or disrupted epidermis and can be spread by picking and biting of the warts. Periungual warts are particularly menacing in a child who is immunosuppressed from organ transplant or cancer chemotherapy (Figure 157).

Clinically, periungual warts are papules and plaques with a rough surface and usually with the appearance of small black dots which represent capillaries in the wart. Onycholysis and nail dystrophy occur if the wart is located in the nail bed and the lateral groove elevates the nail. Treatment of periungual warts in children can be challenging[10–14]. Nearly two-thirds of warts in children disappear within 2 years, so a 'wait and see' approach is reasonable. If the warts are rapidly spreading or otherwise problematic, keratolytic agents such as glutaraldehyde, 15% glycolic acid gel, and formic acid are employed. Liquid nitrogen and lasers have their

proponents, although both can be painful for children. There are mixed reports about the effectiveness of eutectic lidocaine (5% EMLA) in minimizing the discomfort associated with surgical removal of warts in children. The topical sensitizing agent squaric acid dibutylether elicits a cell-mediated immune response when applied to warts in a child who has been previously sensitized. Topical imiquimod, intralesional bleomycin, and oral cimetidine all have their proponents. Efficacy is difficult to assess in warts because there is a high spontaneous resolution rate.

Herpes simplex occurs on the hands in children and is termed a herpetic whitlow. The lesions are tender and vesicular and often follow a cut or break in the skin. The virus can be herpes type 1 or 2. If the diagnosis is not clear, a Tzanck smear or a viral culture can be performed. Treatment is topical or oral nucleoside therapy. Children should be careful not to touch their eyes with the infected fingers to prevent autoinnoculation.

Bacterial infections

Bacterial infections around the nail are not uncommon in children. Blistering distal dactylitis is a *Streptococcal* infection that appears as a non-tender

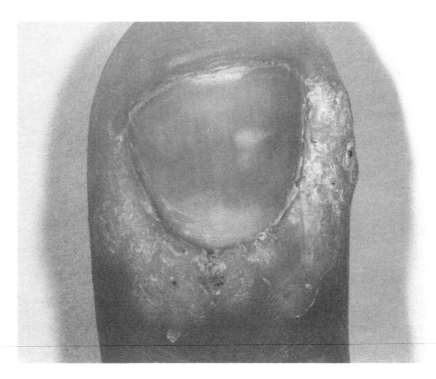

Figure 157 Periungual warts

blister on the distal skin on the volar surface and around the nail. Drainage and penicillin or erythromycin are effective treatments. There are some reports of *Staphylococcus* as the pathogen in blistering distal dactylitis.

Children who suck their fingers or pick at their cuticles are prone to staphylococcal bacterial infections around the nail. Ingrown toenails are often infected and should be cultured so that appropriate antibiotics can be instituted.

Onychomycosis

The prevalence of onychomycosis in children is around 2.6% in one North American study, but

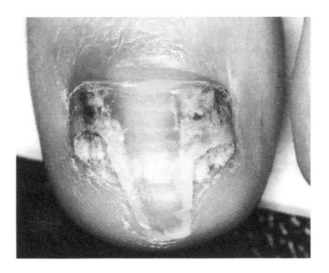

Figure 158 Onychomycosis of the toe

much less than in adults. Typically, the child has a history of tinea pedis and a family history of fungal infections. The most common clinical pattern is distal lateral subungual onychomycosis; *Trichophyton rubrum* is usually the pathogen. The newer antifungal drugs are effective in children and, because the rate of nail growth is faster in children, a shorter duration of therapy is often effective (Figure 158).

Children who suck their fingers are prone to develop candida infections around the nails (Figure 159). Often, these children develop a severe paronychia and are treated with oral antibiotics which can worsen the yeast paronychia. Appropriate topical or oral antifungal treatment usually clears the condition promptly if the child ceases to put his hands in the mouth. Children with chronic mucocutaneous candidiasis or autoimmune polyglandular syndrome have difficulty with recurrent candida onychomycosis[20].

Topical antifungal therapy for onychomycosis in children can be tried as a first-line treatment in mild cases, although the efficacy of topical antifungals is limited. None of the oral antifungal medications are approved for the treatment of onychomycosis in children. There are numerous reports of the safe and effective use of oral antifungal medications in children for onychomycosis[21–23]. Rapid nail growth in children allows for a shorter duration of treatment and excellent response to therapy. Surgical approaches are not commonly used in children (Table 8).

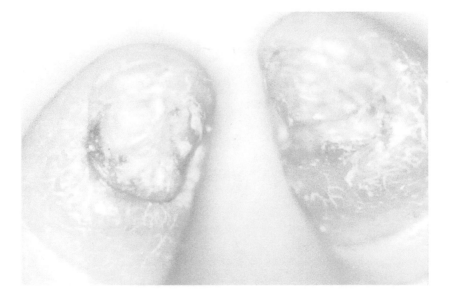

Figure 159 *Candida* infection around the nails caused by finger sucking

PEDIATRIC NAIL TUMORS

The most common benign nail tumor (excluding warts) in children is pyogenic granuloma, a vascular lesion that usually follows trauma or is associated with ingrowing nails (Figure 160). The lesions are red, friable and disturbing to both children and parents because of the ease with which they bleed. The lesions can be cauterized or treated with silver nitrate. If there is any question about the diagnosis, a biopsy should be performed. Pyogenic granuloma can be seen in association with paronychia resulting from isotretinoin therapy in adolescents[24].

Subungual exostosis is a bony subungual growth that is sometimes seen in adolescent children[25]. The lesions often elevate the nail plate and can be tender (Figure 161). Subungual exostosis often follows trauma to the nail. Type I exostosis usually occurs in younger people and is frequently associated with paronychia. X-ray confirms the diagnosis and surgical excision is usually curative[26].

The management of longitudinal pigmented bands in children is a vexing problem[27] (Figure 162). Several reviews suggest that, because melanoma is so rare in children, and because of the risk of general anesthesia and scarring, it may be preferable to

Table 8   Medical treatment of onychomycosis in children. None of the oral fungal medications have FDA approval for the treatment of fungal infections of the nails in children. Adapted from reference 22

Drug	Weight (kg)	Dose	Schedule	Duration	
				Toenails	Fingernails
Griseofulvin	< 50	microsize 15–25 mg/kg/day ultramicrosize 9.9–13.2 mg/kg/day	continuous	26–52 weeks	18–40 weeks
Terbinafine	< 20 20–40 > 40	62.5 q.d. 125 q.d. 250 q.d.	continuous	12 weeks	6 weeks
Itraconazole	< 20 20–40 40–50 > 50	5 mg/kg/day for 1 week/month 100 mg/day for 1 week/month 200 mg/day for 1 week/month 200 mg b.i.d. for 1 week/month	pulse	3 pulses/3 months	2 pulses/2 months
Fluconazole	< 50	3–6 mg/kg/day once weekly	pulse	18–26 weeks	12–16 weeks

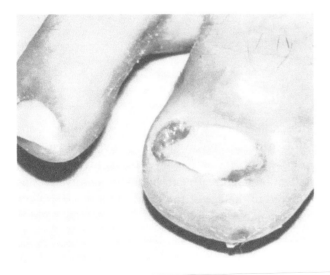

Figure 160 Pyogenic granuloma and granulation tissue associated with ingrown toenail

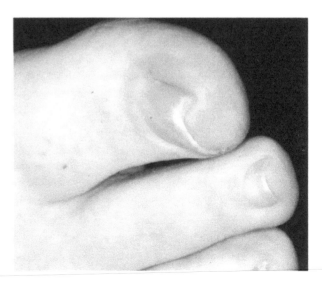

Figure 161 Subungual exostosis

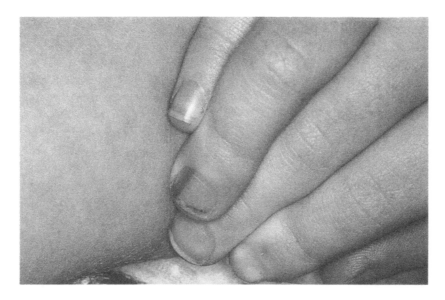

Figure 162 Longitudinal pigmented band

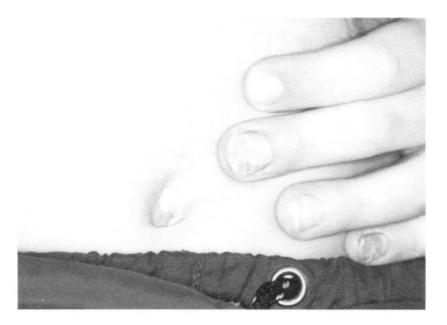

Figure 163 Psoriasis in the umbilicus

simply observe a non-changing pigmented band in a pre-adolescent. Many physicians and parents decide that the risk of scarring is a small price to pay for the reassurance that the pigmented band is not a melanoma, and this is definitely the safest approach.

Psoriasis of the nail in children can be a challenging problem[28]. The diagnosis is sometimes difficult in the absence of cutaneous psoriasis elsewhere on the skin (Figure 163). A family history of psoriasis is often very helpful in establishing the diagnosis. In a large study of 190 children with psoriasis, the presenting site was the scalp in 22% of children, and 36% had nail involvement. Many children with psoriasis of the nails have trachyonychia as the salient finding. Treatment should be conservative and tailored to the age of the child. Topical steroids and tazarotene or calcipiotrene are sometimes helpful. Simple measures, such as avoiding rough or traumatic episodes, minimize the Koebner response.

Parakeratosis pustulosa is a pediatric nail problem that is characterized by nail bed hyperkeratosis, nail plate dystrophy and paronychial inflammation, consisting of scaling and erythema and sometimes pustules. It is characteristically seen in pre-adolescent girls and involves one digit. Tosti and colleagues[29] followed 20 children with parakeratosis pustulosa for an average of 4 years and found a specific diagnosis in 11 of 20 patients. The largest group of eight patients had psoriasis. In four patients, the parakeratosis pustulosa was considered to be a manifestation of allergic contact dermatitis, and atopic dermatitis was suspected in two. Over half of the cases recovered completely. They proposed that parakeratosis pustulosa is a reaction pattern, which can be associated with several dermatologic

conditions and not a single specific nail disease (Figure 164).

Twenty-nail dystrophy of childhood is the name given to the non-specific nail change called trachyonychia[30–32] characterized by pitted nails that are rough and textured. The name twenty-nail dystrophy of childhood is a misnomer because the condition can occur in adults and any number of nails can be affected. In trachyonychia, the surface of the nail plate appears finely etched, giving it a roughened appearance. Trachyonychia occurs in psoriasis, alopecia areata, ichthyosis vulgaris, eczema and other conditions (Figure 165).

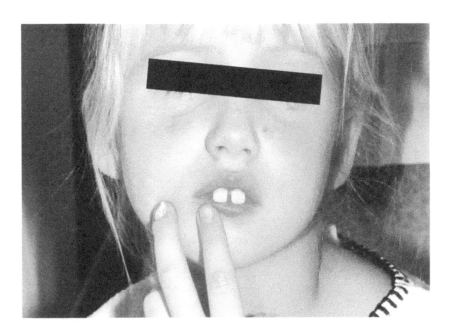

Figure 164 Parakeratosis pustulosa

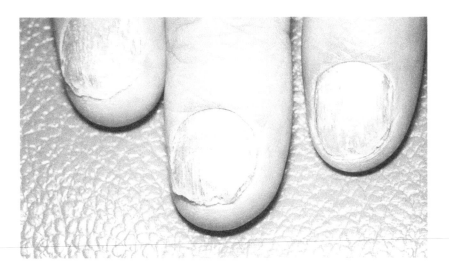

Figure 165 Trachyonychia in a child with lichen planus

Ingrown toenails are a difficult problem at any age, but they can be particularly troublesome with infants and young children[33,34] (Figures 166 and 167). Some newborns have hypertrophied lateral nail folds and/or the fleshy tip of the toe. If the nail becomes embedded, there will be an inflammatory response and often a bacterial infection. Antibiotics and soaks are used when necessary. It is rarely necessary to perform surgery on these toenails but, occasionally, the nail grows into the distal toe pulp. Ingrown nails are sometimes associated with congenital malalignment of the great toenails. In older children, ingrown nails are exacerbated by trimming the nails on an angle. While it might make the nail folds feel better temporarily, the nail spicule will soon regrow into the lateral nail groove and cause pain and potential infection. Treatment should be directed at treating and preventing infection, and education on proper grooming of the toenails. When conservative methods fail, a surgical approach is sometimes necessary. Phenol matricectromy is safe, quick and easy to perform and gives relief quickly[35,36]. The procedure basically removes a thin longitudinal strip of nail from the lateral nail plate. Full-strength phenol is applied to the nail matrix and lateral horns (*see* Chapter 10 for more information). It should only be performed when all else fails.

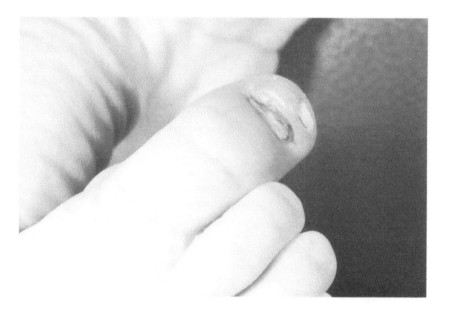

Figure 166 Infant with ingrown toenail

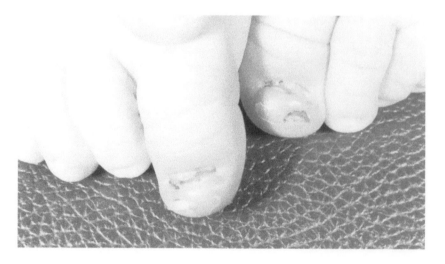

Figure 167 Ingrown toenail

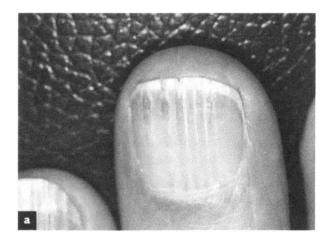

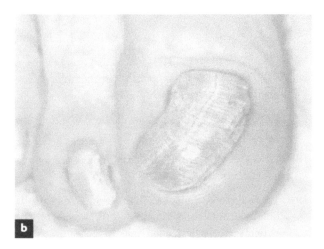

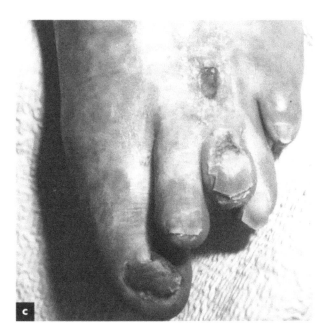

NAIL PROBLEMS IN THE ELDERLY

Potential senile changes of the nails due to advancing age are a decrease in nail growth, change in color from translucent to opaque and yellow, increased thickening and accentuation of longitudinal ridging, and increased brittleness (Figure 168a).

Abnormal biomechanics in the elderly predispose them to a variety of nail problems. Subungual hematoma may occur in the toenails of elderly patients, especially those on anticoagulant therapy, usually in response to trauma or from poorly fitting shoes. Often hammer toes, hallux valgus, and overlapping digits can result in onychogryphosis, onychoclavus (subungual corn), onychauxis (thickened nail plate) (Figure 168b) and onychocryptosis (ingrown nail) (Figure 168c). Onychogryphosis (Figure 169) occurs from neglect and inability of the elderly to groom their nails due to loss of eyesight or the flexibility necessary to reach the toenails. Conservative treatment involves avoidance of tight or poorly fitting shoes and mechanical debridement of severely thickened and onychogryphotic nails. Occasionally, chemical or surgical ablation of the abnormal nail will provide much needed relief for these patients.

A subungual tumor that is sometimes seen in elderly patients is subungual exostosis, a bony nail bed tumor that elevates the nail plate. These benign growths may result from trauma to the nail unit and are frequently painful. These lesions need to be surgically excised (*see* Figures 172 and 173).

Figure 168 Changes from onychorrhexis (a), onychauxis (b) and onychocryptosis (c) in elderly people caused by faulty biomechanics

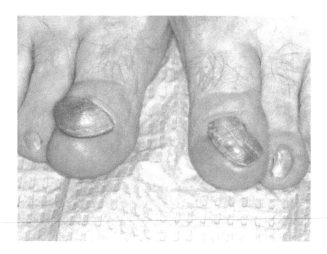

Figure 169 Onychogryphosis in the elderly

Infections

Onychomycosis is more common in the elderly than in younger adults[37-39]. Not all dystrophic nails in the elderly are fungal; in fact only half are. Trauma, psoriasis, lichen planus are all fungus look-alikes in the elderly, so KOH and cultures are important in confirming the diagnosis. Elderly patients may have more difficulty with ambulation, and experience pain due to the thickened unmanageable fungal toenails. Onychomycosis is treated with several modalities: topical, oral and surgical/chemical removal of fungal nails. One topical antifungal medication, cyclopirox lacquer, is approved by the FDA for treatment of onychomycosis. Other topical medications are currently in clinical trials. Oral medications useful for treatment of onychomycosis are griseofulvin, terbinafine, itraconazole, and fluconazole (*see* Table 6 for treatment of onycho-mycosis).

REFERENCES

1. Smith FJ, Coleman CM, Bayoumy NM, Nelson J, McLean D. Novel keratin 17 mutations in pachyony-chia congenita type 2. *J Invest Dermatol* 2001;116:806-8

2. Smith FJ, Morley Sm, Mclean WH. A novel connexin 30 mutation in Clouston syndrome. *J Invest Dermatol* 2002;118:530-2

3. Baran R. Congenital malalignment of the toenail. *Arch Dermatol* 1980;116:1346

4. Baran R, Grognard C, Duhard E, Drape JL. Congenital malalignment of the great toenail: an enigma resolved by a new surgical treatment. *Br J Dermatol* 1998;139:72

5. DeBerker D. What do Beau's lines mean? *Int J Dermatol* 1994;33:545-6

6. Bernier V, Labreze C, Bury F, Taieb A. Nail matrix arrest in the course of hand, foot and mouth disease. *Eur J Pediatr* 2001;160:649-51

7. Tosti A, Piraccini BM, Camacho-Martinez F. Onychomadesis and pyogenic granuloma following cast immobilization. *Arch Dermatol* 2001;137:231-2

8. Wester JP, Van Eps RS, Stopughamer A, Girbes AR. Critical illness onychomadesis. *Intensive Care Med* 2000;26:1698-700

9. Karo DL, Cohen BA. Onychodystrophy in lichen striatus. *Pediatr Dermatol* 1993;10:359-61

10. Meineke V, Reichrath, J, Reinhold U. Verrucae vulgaris in children: successful simulated X-ray treat-ment (a suggestion-based therapy). *Dermatology* 2002;204:287-9

11. Grussendorf-Conen EI, Jacobs S. Efficacy of imiquimod 5% cream in the treatment of recalcitrant warts in children. *Pediatr Dermatol* 2002;19:263-6

12. Torrelo A. What's new in the treatment of viral warts in children. *Pediatr Dermatol* 2002;19:191-9

13. Sparling JD, Checketts SR, Chaoman MS. Imiquimod for plantar and periungual warts. *Cutis* 2001;68:397-9

14. Tosti A, Piraccini BM. Warts of the nail unit: surgical and non surgical approaches. *Dermatol Surg* 2001;27:235-9

15. Cengizlier R, Uysal G, Guvan A, Tulek N. Herpetic finger infection. *Cutis* 2002;69:291-2

16. Whitley JR. Herpes simplex virus in children. *Curr Treat Options Neurol* 2002;4:231-7

17. Rhody C. Bacterial infections of the skin. *Prim Care* 2000;27:459-73

18. Prose NS, Mayer FE. Bacterial skin infections in adolescents. *Adolesc Med* 1990;1:325-32

19. Woroszylski A, Duran C, Tamayo L, Orozoco ML. Staphylococcal blistering dactylitis: report of two patients. *Pediatr Dermatol* 1996;13:292-3

20. Manz B, Scholz GH, Willgerodt H, Haustein UF, Nenoff P. Autoimmune polyglandular syndrome (APS) type 1 and candida onychomycosis. *Eur J Dermatol* 2002;12:283-6

21. Gupta A, Sibbald RG, Lynde CW, Hull PR, Prussick R, Shcer NH. Onychomycosis in children: preva-lence and treatment strategies. *J Am Acad Dermatol* 1997;36:395-402

22. Huang PH, Paller AS. Itraconazole pulse therapy for dermatophyte onychomycosis in children. *Arch Pediatr Adolesc Med* 2000;154:614-18

23. Farkas B, Paul C, Dobozy A, Hunyada J. Terbinafine (Lamisil) treatment of toenail onychomycosis in patients with insulin-dependent and non-insulin-dependent diabetes mellitus: a multicentre trial. *Br J Dermatol* 2002;146:254-60

24. Blumenthal G. Paronychia and pyogenic granuloma-like lesions with isotretinoin. *J Am Acad Dermatol* 1984;10:677-8

25. Biermann JS. Common benign lesions of bone in children and adolescents. *J Pediatr Orthop* 2002;22:268-73

26. Lokiec F, Ezra E, Krasin E, Keret D, Weintraub S. Simple and efficient surgical technique for subungual exostosis. *J Pediatr Orthop* 2001;21:76–9

27. Goettmann-Bonvallot S, Andre J, Baelaich S. Longitudinal melanonychia in children: a clinical and histopathologic study of 40 cases. *J Am Acad Dermatol* 1999;41:17–22

28. Al Fourzan AS, Nanda A. A survey of childhood psoriasis in Kuwait. *Pediatr Dermatol* 1994;11:116–19

29. Tosti A, Peluso AM, Zucchelli V. Clinical features and long-term follow-up of 20 cases of parakeratosis pustulosa. *Pediatr Dermatol* 1998;15:259–63

30. Joshi RK, Abanmi A, Ohman SG, Heleem A. Lichen planus of the nails presenting as trachyonychia. *Int J Dermatol* 1993;32:54–5

31. Tosti A, Fanti PA, Morellim R, Bardazzi F. Spongiotic trachyonychia. *Arch Dermatol* 1991;127:584–5

32. Tosti A , Piraccini BM, Cambiaaghi S, Jorizzo M. Nail lichen planus in children: clinical features, response to treatment, and long-term follow-up. *Arch Dermatol* 2001;137:1027–32

33. Piraccini BM, Parente GL, Varotti E, Tosti A. Congenital hypertrophy of the lateral nail folds of the hallux: clinical features and follow-up of seven cases. *Pediatr Dermatol* 2000;17:348–51

34. Honig PJ. After effects of congenital ingrown toenails. *Pediatr Dermatol* 2001;18:454

35. Bostanci S, Ekmekci P, Gurgy E. Chemical matricectomy with phenol for the treatment of ingrowing toenail: a review of the literature and follow-up of 172 treated patients. *Acta Derm Venereol* 2001;81:181–3

36. Pappert AS, Scher RK, Cohen JL. Nail disorders in children. *Pediatr Clin North Am* 1991;38:921–40

37. Martin ES, Elewski BE. Cutaneous fungal infections in the elderly. *Clin Geriatr Med* 2002;18:59–75

38. Scherer WP, McCreary JP, Hayes WW. The diagnosis of onychomycosis in a geriatric population: a study of 450 cases in South Florida. *J Am Podiatr Med Assoc* 2001;91:456–64

39. Scher RK. Onychomycosis: a significant medical disorder. *J Am Acad Dermatol* 1996;35:52–5

9

Nail tumors

Tumors can occur in any part of the nail unit. Nail tumors can be identified by clinical presentation, X-ray findings and biopsy. Both benign and malignant lesions of the nail are seen.

BENIGN TUMORS

There are several types of fibroma (Figures 170 and 171) that occur around the nail.

Koenen's tumors

Koenen's tumors are asymptomatic tumors that occur in adolescence in patients with tuberous sclerosis. They are often multiple and can cause depressions in the nail plate. Surgery is the treatment for bothersome lesions. Acquired digital fibrokeratomas are small growths that appear around the nail and are fleshy, asymptomatic and may have a keratotic distal tip.

Subungual exostosis

Subungual exostosis is not a true tumor but rather a bony outgrowth that occurs under the nail and elevates the nail plate[1,2] (Figures 172 and 173). They are more frequent on the toes and usually follow trauma. Exostoses exhibit the triad of a bony growth under the nail, radiographic changes and pain. Type I exostosis is more common in females and the typical age of occurrence is during the second and third decades. X-ray is mandatory. The treatment for subungual exostosis is surgical excision.

Glomus tumor

A glomus tumor is a painful lesion in the nail bed[3,4]. It is usually visible through the nail plate as a red or blue macule, although, when involving the matrix, it may not be visible (Figure 174). There may be over-

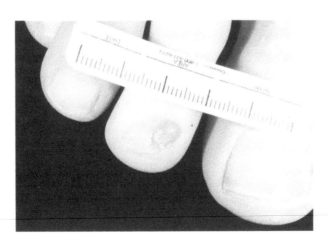

Figure 170 Fibroma of the nail fold

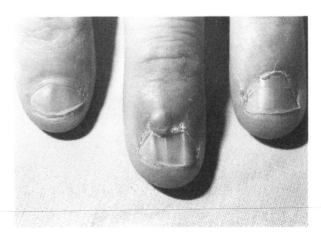

Figure 171 Fibroma causing nail plate grooves

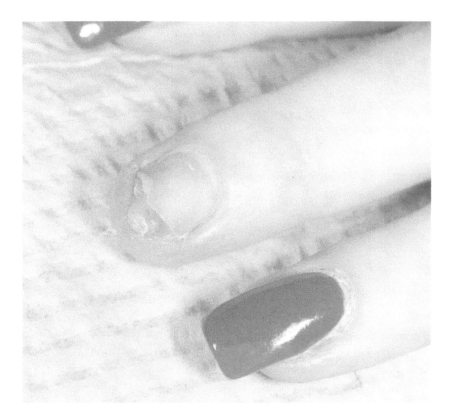

Figure 172 Subungual exostosis of the finger, elevating the nail plate

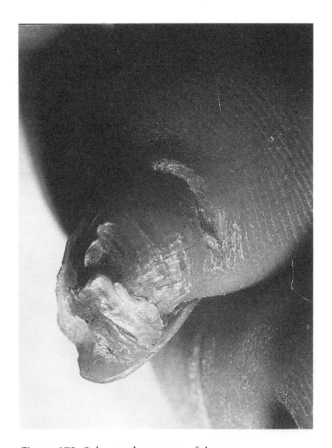

Figure 173 Subungual exostosis of the toe

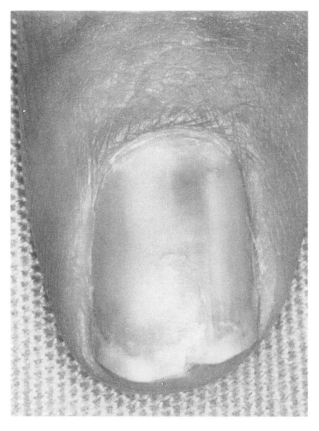

Figure 174 Glomus tumor of the nail bed

lying thinning of the nail plate. The cause of glomus tumors is not known, but often there is a history of trauma to the affected digit. The patient describes intense pinpoint pain with throbbing, and the pain is often exacerbated by pressure or cold temperature. The treatment of choice is surgical excision.

Pyogenic granuloma

A pyogenic granuloma is a benign tumor that usually follows injury to the paronychial or subungual area.

The lesion is usually red, bleeds easily due to the exuberant quality of the granulation tissue, and may be friable, eroded or crusted (Figures 175 and 176). Histological diagnosis is important because the differential diagnosis includes amelanotic melanoma.

Onychomatricoma

Onychomatricoma (Figure 177) is a nail tumor that is characterized by longitudinal yellow bands and

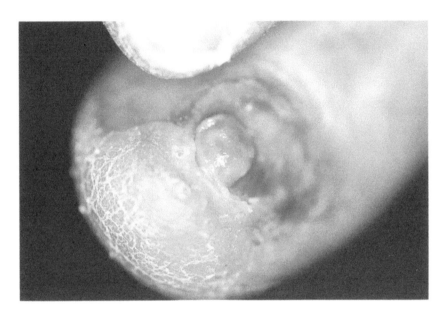

Figure 175 Pyogenic granuloma

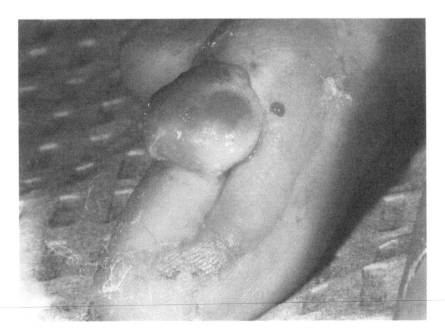

Figure 176 Pyogenic granuloma of the nail following trauma

ridging. This consists of a group of hollow channels in a funnel-shaped configuration.

Myxoid pseudocyst

Myxoid pseudocysts, also called digital mucous cysts or synovial cysts, are found most commonly on the terminal digits of the fingers (Figure 178). Rarely, they develop on the toes (Figure 179). They typically present as non-inflamed, solitary, skin-colored or bluish nodules under a centimeter in size. Most are not painful, but tenderness may develop if the cyst is traumatized. The nodules are not true cysts but are formed by focal accumulations of mucin in the dermis, without a defined lining or cyst wall. Therefore, some clinicians refer to these lesions as pseudocysts. They are filled with a clear, viscous, sticky, mucinous fluid (Figure 180). When the cyst occurs at the proximal nail fold, a depressed groove in the nail plate may form along the entire length of

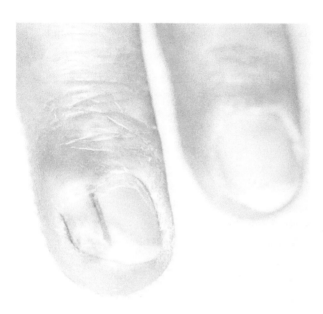

Figure 177 Onychomatricomas, characterized by longitudinal yellow bands and ridging of the nail

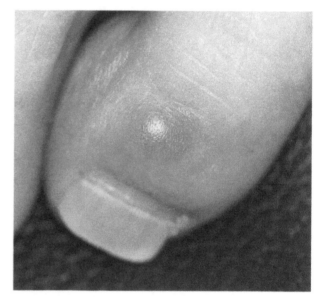

Figure 179 Myxoid pseudocyst on the toe

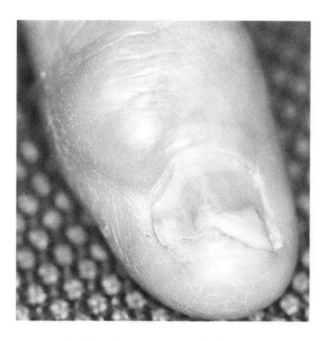

Figure 178 Myxoid pseudocyst on the finger

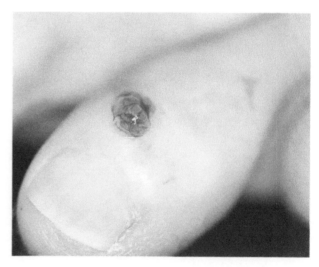

Figure 180 Mucinous fluid in a myxoid pseudocyst

the nail surface (Figure 181). Women are more commonly affected than men and osteoarthritis is sometimes present in the adjacent joint, but it is unclear why these associations exist.

Researchers do not agree on the pathogenesis of digital mucous cysts. One theory is that mucin accumulates – either spontaneously or due to trauma – in areas near but not connected with the joint space. Another theory is that there is a connection from the joint space to the cyst, with extrusion of mucin from the joint to the nodule. Proponents of this theory may refer to the entity as a synovial cyst.

MALIGNANT TUMORS

Squamous cell carcinoma

Squamous cell carcinoma of the nail is not rare, but, fortunately, rarely metastasizes. It is seen most commonly in the sixth to seventh decade of life and can present as paronychia, onycholysis with hyperkeratosis (Figures 182 and 183), or pyoderma. Squamous cell carcinoma can be associated with radiation exposure and with human papilloma virus (HPV) infection, particularly HPV types 16, 18, 34 and 35. Moh's surgery is the treatment of choice (Figure 184).

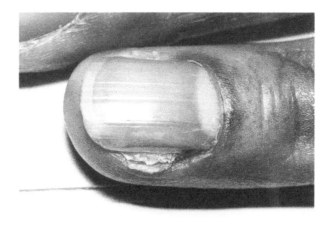

Figure 182 Squamous cell carcinoma of the nail, with onycholysis

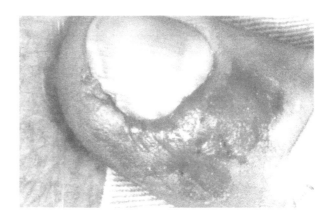

Figure 183 Squamous cell carcinoma *in situ* in the nail fold

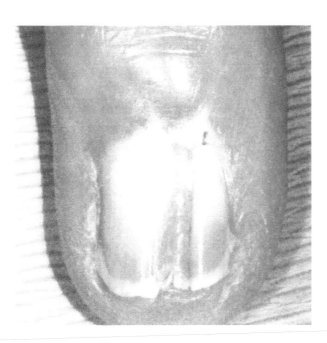

Figure 181 Mucous cyst with longitudinal groove in the nail plate

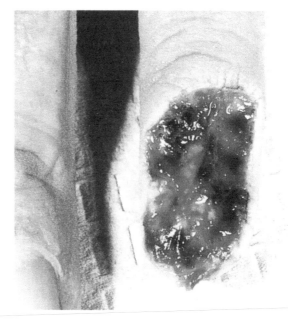

Figure 184 Squamous cell carcinoma after treatment with Moh's surgery

Keratoacanthoma

Keratoacanthoma (Figure 185) is a rapidly growing, painful subungual nail tumor that can erode the bone and cause a radiolucency on X-ray. Keratoacanthoma is more common in men than women and occurs in the age group of 30–60 years. Moh's surgery is usually curative, although, in advanced bone invasion, amputation is sometimes performed. Diagnosis may be made by clinical features, X-ray and histology.

Longitudinal melanonychia

Longitudinal melanonychia or melanonychia striata longitudinalis is a pigmented band of the nail extending from the nail matrix to the free edge of the nail plate. Pigmented bands in the nail have many causes, the most important of which is melanoma. The diagnosis of nail melanoma[4-11] is often difficult, based on clinical features alone; however, widening or darkening or variegated color of the band, location on first or second digit, and the presence of pigment on the

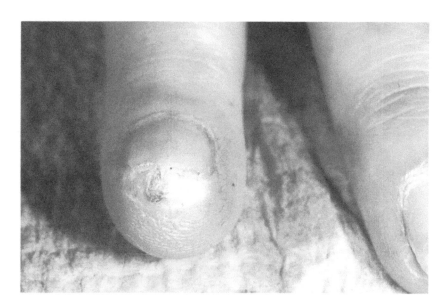

Figure 185 Keratoacanthoma of the nail bed

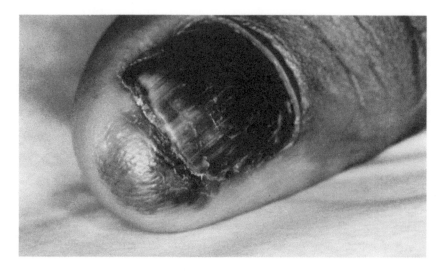

Figure 186 Malignant melanoma of the nail

Table 10 Mnemonic for clinical diagnosis of melanoma of the nail: the ABC rule. Adapted from reference 12

A	Age: the peak age of incidence of nail melanoma is in the 5th–7th decade
B	Brown, black and breadth of > 3 mm in width of band
C	Change in the morphology of the nail or lack of change after treatment
D	Digit most commonly involved: thumb and great toenail
E	Extension of pigment onto nail fold (Hutchinson's sign)
F	Family or personal history of melanoma or dysplastic nevus

nail folds (Hutchinson's sign) are all worrisome features (Figure 186). If the diagnosis of nail melanoma in an adult is considered, a biopsy is mandatory (Table 10). In a Caucasian adult, any newly formed pigmented band usually mandates biopsy.

Longitudinal melanonychia can be due to melanin synthesis from usually dormant melanocytes, or an increase in the number of melanocytes. Longitudinal melanonychia arises in a number of benign situations. Benign pigmented bands are common in darkly pigmented people.

REFERENCES

1. Lokiec F, Ezra E, Krasin E, Keret D, Weintraub S. A simple and efficient surgical technique for subungual exostosis. *J Pediatr Orthop* 2001;21:76–9

2. Wang TC, Wu YH, Su HY. Subungual exostosis. *J Dermatol* 1999;26:72–4

3. Takata H, Ikunta Y, Ishida O, Kimori K. Treatment of subungual glomus tumour. *Hand Surg* 2001;6:25–7

4. Alam M, Scher RK. Current topics in nail surgery. *J Cutan Med Surg* 1999;3:324–35

5. Fleckman P, Omura EF. Histopathology of the nail. *Adv Dermatol* 2001;17:385–406

6. Kawabae Y, Ohara K, Hino H, Tamaki K. Two kinds of Hutchinson's sign, benign and malignant. *J Am Acad Dermatol* 2001;44:305–7

7. Grunwald MH, Yerushalmi J, Glesinger R, Lapid O, Zirkin HU. Subungual amelanotic melanoma. *Cutis* 2000;65:303–4

8. Banfield CC, Dawber RP. Nail melanoma: a review of the literature with recommendations to improve patient management. *Br J Dermatol* 1999;141:628–32

9. Mohrle M, Hafner HM. Is subungual melanoma related to trauma? *Dermatology* 2002;204:259–61

10. Clarkson JH, McAllister RM, Cliff SH, Powell B. Subungual melanoma *in situ*: two independent streaks in one nail bed. *Br J Plast Surg* 2002;55:165–7

11. Speren JM. Malignant tumors of the nail unit. *Dermatol Ther* 2002;15:124

12. Levi EK, Kagen MH, Scher RK, Grossman M, Altman E. The ABC rule for clinical detection of subungual melanoma. *J Am Acad Dermatol* 2000;42:269–74

10

Nail surgery

The major objectives of nail surgery are to diagnose ambiguous nail conditions and to remove painful or disfiguring nail lesions. The prerequisites for successful nail surgery are adequate anesthesia and hemostasis, knowledge of surgical anatomy and the physiology of the nail, and proper technique. In addition, mycology to rule out fungal infection, X-rays when a nail tumor is suspected, and photographs of the nail prior to surgery are important. A full PAR (procedure, alternatives, risks) conference should explain the potential for scarring, infection, bleeding, and pain.

Three important concepts in the anatomy and physiology of the nail unit should be understood prior to nail surgery.

(1) The nail matrix is responsible for the formation of the nail plate and thus damage to the matrix could result in a permanent nail dystrophy. The proximal matrix forms the superficial part of the nail plate and the distal matrix forms the inferior part of the nail plate. It is preferable to biopsy the distal matrix rather than the proximal matrix because any defect would be on the inferior surface of the nail plate and not be visible.

(2) There is no subcutaneous tissue associated with the nail unit; therefore, the dermis of the nail bed in the matrix sits directly on the periostium of the distal digit. Biopsy specimens in the nail bed and nail matrix are taken down to bone.

(3) The location of the extensor tendon of the digit is about 12 mm proximal to the cuticle and must be respected in extensive nail surgery.

Perfect anesthesia is important for patient acceptance of nail surgery. A digital block and/or a wing block (Figure 187) is performed by injecting a small

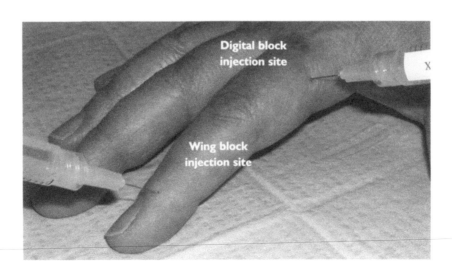

Figure 187 Injection sites for wing block (left) and digital block (right)

amount of plain lidocaine at the base of the digit on the lateral sides or in the proximal/lateral nail folds, respectively. A tourniquet is not often needed but, when one is used, a flat Penrose drain is best. Hemostasis can be achieved by pressing on the lateral digital arteries on the sides of the digit during the procedure.

Several instruments make nail surgery easier: a Freer septum elevator, double-action nail nipper, and an English nail splitter are useful additions to the standard dermatologic surgery instruments (Figure 188).

The fundamental procedures upon which other nail surgeries are built are nail avulsion and matrix exploration. Nail avulsion involves loosening the nail plate from the nail bed, matrix and nail folds and then lifting it off the nail bed (Figure 189)[1]. For a matrix exploration, releasing incisions are made at the angle of the proximal and lateral nail fold (Figure 190). The proximal nail fold is reflected back so that

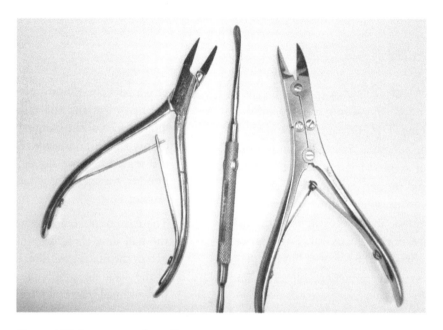

Figure 188 Instruments for nail surgery

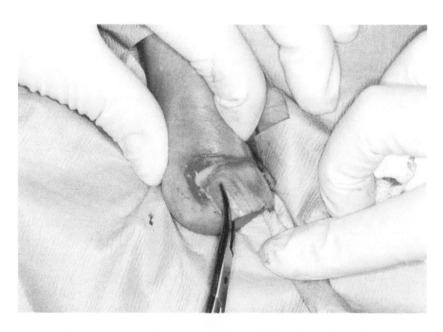

Figure 189 Nail avulsion by loosening the nail plate from the nail bed, matrix and folds and lifting the plate off the bed

the matrix is visible. Subsequently, a punch biopsy or elliptical excision of a tumor can be performed as indicated. At the end of the procedure, the nail fold is returned to its normal position and sutures or steri strips are used to secure it in place (Figure 191).

The type of nail procedure performed depends on the location of the pathology, the size and nature of the lesion, and always with consideration for the final cosmetic outcome. For a small nail bed or nail matrix lesion, a punch biopsy will adequately sample the lesion and often remove it; the punch can be performed after nail avulsion or through the intact nail plate (Figure 192). An elliptical excision of the nail bed should be oriented in the longitudinal direction whereas an ellipse in the matrix is oriented in the horizontal direction (Figures 193 and 194).

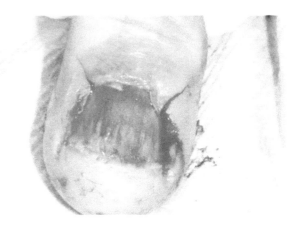

Figure 191 Proximal nail fold replaced and sutured with steri strips

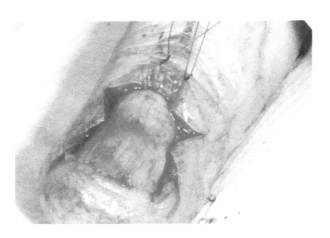

Figure 190 Matrix exploration performed by reflecting the proximal nail fold

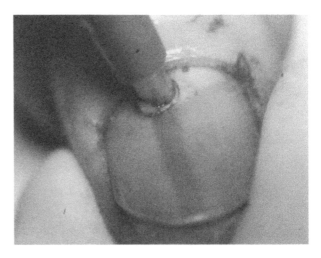

Figure 192 Punch biopsy can be taken through the nail plate into the nail bed or nail matrix

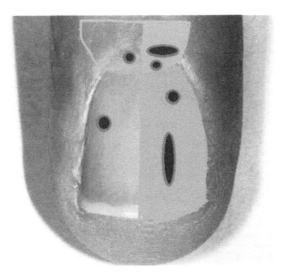

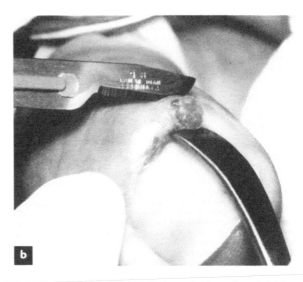

Figure 193 (a) In a lateral longitudinal nail biopsy, a longitudinal section is removed, including the lateral nail fold, nail matrix, nail bed and hyponychium. (b) Biopsy of the proximal nail fold is performed to remove a space-occupying lesion of the nail fold. The resultant defect heals neatly by secondary intention

Sutures should be placed to approximate wound edges in larger excisions for the best cosmetic outcome. Handle and orient the specimen carefully so that the pathologist can obtain the optimal results.

Ingrown toenails are painful and do not always respond to conservative measures (Figure 195). The simplest surgical management of ingrown toenails and pincer nails is phenol matricectomy[2-4]. In this procedure, a longitudinal portion of the lateral nail plate is removed (Figures 196 and 197). Full-strength phenol 88% is applied several times with a small cotton swab to the lateral horn of the nail matrix and then the area is neutralized with alcohol or saline. The phenol denatures the protein of the matrix and prevents regrowth of the nail plate in that area. The nail folds and nail bed should be protected from the phenol. There is usually drainage for several weeks after the procedure, but the nail usually heals with a narrower nail plate that has a satisfactory esthetic appearance (Figure 198).

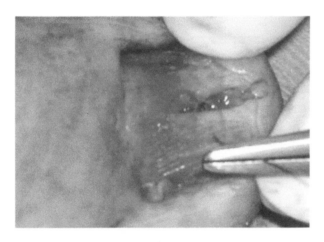

Figure 194 A longitudinal surgical defect resulting from excision of a nail bed lesion can be repaired with absorbable suture

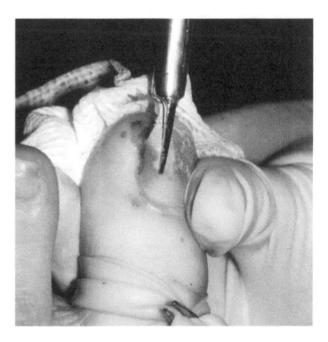

Figure 196 Removal of longitudinal portion of the lateral nail plate in surgical management of ingrown toenail and pincer nail

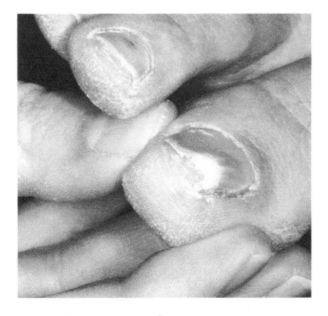

Figure 195 Ingrown toenails

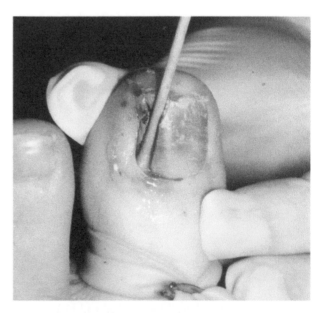

Figure 197 Application of full-strength phenol to lateral horn of nail matrix

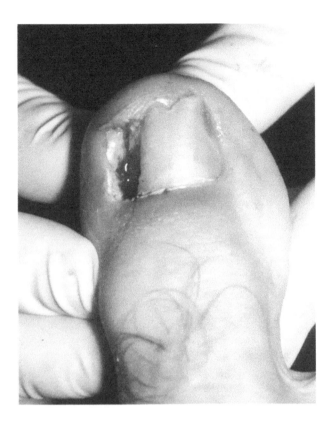

Figure 198 Healed nail, with narrower nail plate

COMPLICATIONS OF NAIL SURGERY

When the basic principles of nail surgery are followed, nail surgery is a safe procedure with an acceptable cosmetic outcome. Most of the complications of nail surgery are related to infection and scarring. Aseptic technique is important in preparing the patient for nail surgery. Prophylactic antibiotics are usually not necessary, except in patients with prosthetic heart valves or where there is a suspicion of infection. Scarring is a potential complication of nail surgery involving the nail matrix, the structure responsible for forming the nail plate. When possible, biopsy specimens from the nail matrix should be taken from the distal part of the matrix to minimize a split nail. Mid-line biopsies also have a higher rate of scarring so, if given a choice, the biopsy of the lateral matrix is less risky than mid-line nail biopsy.

Less common complications of nail surgery include reflect sympathic dystrophy following nail surgery and the formation of pyogenic granuloma.

REFERENCES

1. Daniel CR III. Basic nail plate avulsion. *J Dermatol Surg Oncol* 1992;18:685–8

2. Gerritsma-Bleeker CL, Klaase JM, Geelkerken RH, Hermans J, van Det RJ. Partial matrix excision or segmental phenolization for ingrowing toenails. *Arch Surg* 2002;137:320–5

3. Herold N, Houdhisn S, Riegels-Nielsen P. A prospective comparison of wedge matrix resection with nail matrix phenolization for the treatment of ingrown toenail. *J Foot Ankle Surg* 2001;40:390–5

4. Bostanci S, Ekmekci P, Gurgey E. Chemical matricectomy with phenol for the treatment of ingrowing toenail: a review of the literature and follow-up of 172 treated patients. *Acta Derm Venereol* 2001;81:181–3

FURTHER READING

Baran R, Hanneke E, Richert B. Pincer nails: definition and surgical treatment. *J Derm Surg* 2001;27:261

Moossavi M, Scher RK. Complications of nail surgery: a review of the literature. *J Derm Surg* 2001;27:225–8

Fleckman P. Surgical anatomy of the nail. *Derm Surg* 2001;20:257

11

Nail cosmetics

Well-groomed nails are an important fashion accessory for the modern woman. Americans spent over 6 billion dollars on nail salon services in 2000. While nail cosmetics are used safely by millions of women, there are some problems associated with their use. The problems associated with nail cosmetics fall into one of four categories: allergic, irritant, mechanical and infectious. Recognition of nail cosmetic problems and substitution of alternative products and techniques can help women continue to use nail cosmetics safely (Table 11).

Allergic reactions to nail cosmetics occur with several categories of products: acrylates in sculptured nails and photo-polymerized gel nail extensions,

formaldehyde in nail hardeners, toluene sulfonamide formaldehyde resin in some nail enamels, and nickel in the metal beads in nail polishes (not commonly used but present in some older polishes). Allergic reactions to nail products present as itching, burning and stinging around the nail and often on the eyelids following the nail procedure (Figure 199). The nails may show onycholysis, nail bed hyperkeratosis (Figure 200) and paronychial erythema and scale (Figure 201). Patch testing will usually provide the diagnosis and allow the physician to suggest alternative products (Figure 202). Methylmethacrylate is the most potent ingredient in acrylic nail polishes

Table 11   Potential problems with nail cosmetics

Risk of infection (usually following trauma)
Bacteria
Fungal
Viral

Allergic
Methylmethacrylate
Toluene sulfonamide formaldehyde resin
Cyanoacrylate glue
Nickel in beads in nail enamel

Irritant reaction
Cuticle remover
Nail polish removers (acetone, acetate)
Water and detergents
Yellow-staining of the nail from dark polish
Keratin granulations from prolonged use of nail enamel

Mechanical/traumatic injury
Instrument damage to cuticle and nails
Mechanical damage from long nail extensions

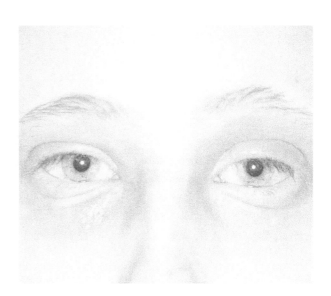

Figure 199 Allergic reactions to nail products on the eyelids from toluene sulfonamide formaldehyde resin in nail enamel used in salons. Many nail polishes in department stores and drug stores are free of this substance

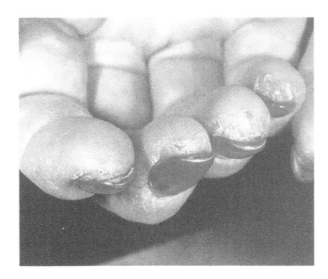

Figure 200 Itching, scaling and hyperkeratosis, with inflammation follow from allergic reaction to methyl-methacrylate in acrylic nail polishes

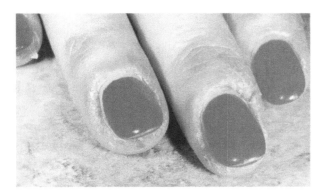

Figure 201 Allergic reaction to acrylate showing parony-chial inflammation following acrylic nail polish application

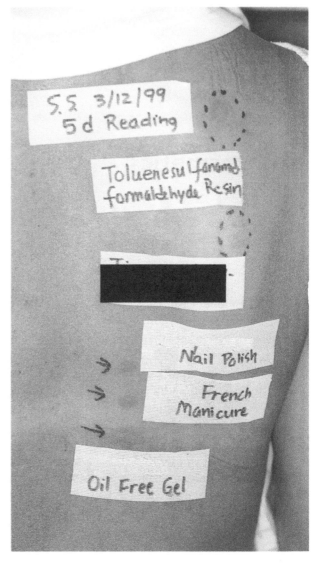

Figure 202 Patch testing of nail cosmetics

and is used more in unlicensed salons because it is less costly than safer ethylmethacrylate.

Irritant reactions occur when nail product and services expose the nail unit to irritating products. Cuticle remover, acetone and acetate in nail polish remover, and even soapy water can act as contact irritants and predispose to onycholysis and paronychia. Brittle nails and onychoschizia can result from excessive use of irritating substances used in manicures (Figure 203). Brightly colored or dark nail enamel used continuously can result in yellow staining of the nail plate due to yellow dye present in many nail polish formulations (Figure 204).

Infections related to nail products can be bacterial, fungal or viral. Mechanical and infectious

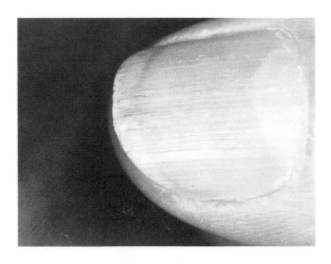

Figure 203 Brittle nails exacerbated by nail cosmetics

problems arising from nail products and services are often related to cutting or clipping the cuticle. Clipping the cuticle can result in cuts in the skin that allow bacteria and yeast to gain access to the nail unit and cause acute and chronic paronychia. Infections can be transmitted from person to person by inadequately sterilized instruments (Figure 205). Items that cannot be sanitized, such as files, should be discarded after each use to avoid transmission of warts, fungus and bacteria. Sharp instruments used to clean under the nail plate and push back the cuticle can trigger oncholysis and paronychia.

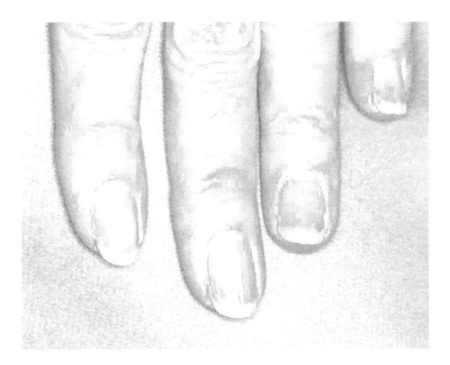

Figure 204 Yellow staining of the nail plate due to yellow dye present in nail polish

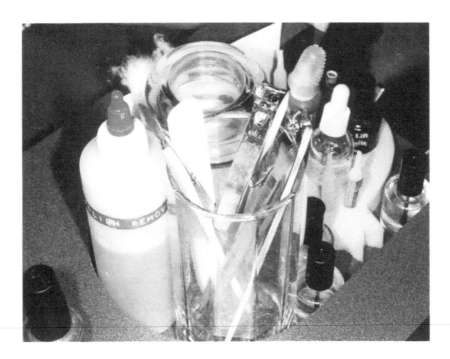

Figure 205 Salon instruments not properly sterilized

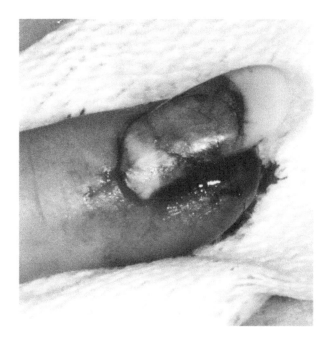

Figure 206 Trauma due to long nail extensions

Table 12 Guidelines for patients to assure safe use of nail cosmetics and salon services

1. Be sure your salon and nail technician are licensed

2. Ask how the implements and footbaths are sterilized. Better still, purchase your own instruments and take them with you each time

3. Do not allow your cuticles to be cut

4. If you experience any burning or stinging after a salon service, you may be having an allergic reaction; remove the product as soon as possible

5. If you suspect that methylmethacrylate (MMA) is being used, ask about it and/or report it

6. If you use artificial nail enhancements, keep them short

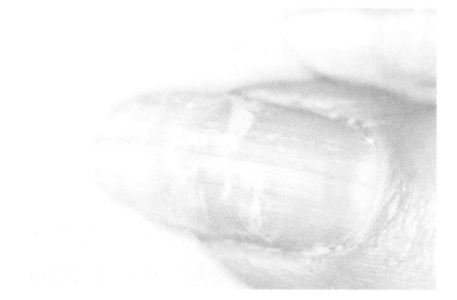

Figure 207 Nail keratin granulations caused by nail enamel

Nails, artificial or natural, that are too long will cause excessive force on the nail bed and can result in onycholysis and nail trauma (Figure 206). Long-term use of nail enamel can cause white friable areas on the nail plate, termed nail keratin granulations (Figure 207). Table 12 provides guidelines for patients to ensure that nail cosmetics and salon services are used wisely and safely.

FURTHER READING

Moossavi M, Scher RK. Nail care products. *Clin Dermatol* 2001;19:445–8

Draelos ZD. Nail cosmetic issues. *Dermatol Clin* 2000; 18:675–83

Guin JD. Eyelid dermatology from methacrylates used for nail enhancements. *Contact Dermatitis* 1998;39:312–13

Index

For Product Safety Concerns and Information please contact our EU representative GPSR@taylorandfrancis.com Taylor & Francis Verlag GmbH, Kaufingerstraße 24, 80331 München, Germany

T - #0073 - 160425 - C0 - 279/216/7 [9] - CB - 9781850705956 - Gloss Lamination